Living Well

with

HIV and AIDS

Third Edition

Living Well
with
HIV and AIDS

Third Edition

Allen L. Gifford, M.D.

Kate Lorig, R.N., Dr.P.H.

Diana Laurent, M.P.H.

Virginia González, M.P.H.

BULL PUBLISHING COMPANY
BOULDER, COLORADO

Bull Publishing Company
P.O. Box 1377
Boulder, CO 80306
(800) 676-2855
www.bullpub.com

ISBN: 978-0-923521-86-8

Publisher: James Bull
Managing Editor: Erin Mulligan
Developmental Editor: Lynn Gordon
Interior Design and Production: Shadow Canyon Graphics
Cover Design: Lightbourne Images

LIBRARY OF CONGRESS CATALOGING-IN-PUBLICATION DATA

LIVING WELL WITH HIV & AIDS / ALLEN L. GIFFORD . . . [ET AL.]. 3RD ED.
    P. CM
    INCLUDES BIBLIOGRAPHICAL REFERENCES AND INDEX.
    ISBN 0-923521-86-O
    1. AIDS (DISEASE)—POPULAR WORKS. I. TITLE: LIVING WELL WITH
HIV AND AIDS. III. GIFFORD, ALLEN L.

RC607.A26 L587 2000
362.1'969792—DC21   00-023029

CONTENTS

ACKNOWLEDGMENTS

This book was produced with the help of many people. None, however, deserve greater appreciation or more acknowledgment than the many people with HIV/AIDS, and their friends, families, and loved ones, who have brought their own life-experiences to bear, and have made suggestions about things to include in this book, and ways to improve it. Doctors, nurses, health educators, and other health professionals who have devoted themselves to improving the lives of people with HIV/AIDS have all contributed many of the ideas included here.

This work would not be possible without the generous support of the U.S. Veterans Health Administration, the VA Quality Enhancement Research Initiative for HIV, the Stanford Patient Education Research Center, and the Robert Wood Johnson Foundation.

We owe a great debt to the hard work of our editors, Erin Mulligan and Lynn Gordon. Without their efforts this project would not have been possible. Certain other important individuals deserve special mention. Chris Adams helped conceive and plan this project, and his intelligence, wit, irreverence, and bravery in facing his own illness inspired us all. Vivian Vestal was for many years our very dear friend and the very best and most dedicated of our peer-leaders in the Positive Self-Management Program for HIV. Janet Tobacman and Joe DiMilia of Kaiser Permanente Northern California have been invaluable and tireless in their support for this book, and for the Positive Self-Management Program for over a decade. Special thanks are also due to Halsted Holman, Samuel Bozzette, Marian Minor, David Sobel, Janet Tobacman, Joe DiMilia, Jill Bormann, Marty Shively, and all the extraordinary nurses, staff, and physicians who care for for people with HIV at the VA San Diego Healthcare System, the University of California – San Diego, and the University of California – San Francisco.

To Chris Adams and Vivian Vestal

HOW TO USE THIS BOOK

No one wants to have HIV or AIDS. But just because you have HIV/AIDS* doesn't mean that your life comes to an end. This book has been written to help people with HIV/ AIDS learn a healthy way to live. This may sound strange. How can one have an illness and live a healthy life at the same time? To answer this question, it is important to think about what "health" really is: *Health is soundness of body and mind, and a healthy life is a life which seeks that soundness.* A healthy way to live with any illness is to work at overcoming the physical, emotional, and social problems caused by the illness. The goal is to achieve the greatest possible physical capability and pleasure from life. People with all kinds of illnesses do this successfully every day. This is what this book is all about.

But can people with HIV/AIDS live healthy lives? Of course. HIV/AIDS is a chronic disease like many others. It has many similarities to conditions such as diabetes and heart disease, to name just two. For people with HIV/AIDS, there are more treatments and programs available now than ever before. If HIV/AIDS becomes symptomatic, it causes decreased function of the immune system. The chronic symptoms that may result can cause people to lose physical conditioning. In addition, these symptoms may cause feelings of emotional distress, such as depression, frustration, and helplessness. All these things can affect how life is lived. The job of the person living with HIV/AIDS is to find ways to deal with these symptoms and decrease the effects of HIV on

---

* The terminology used in discussing HIV-related disease is clumsy. We don't want to use just the term *AIDS* because this word excludes all people with HIV infection who don't have an AIDS diagnosis. Therefore, throughout the book we use the term *HIV/AIDS* to refer in general to the full range of conditions caused by HIV infection.

life. To do this well, you need to be involved in planning and decision making about how you're going to live with your illness. You need to be a *self-manager*.

You will not find any miracles or cures in these pages. Rather, you will find tips, ideas, and resources about how to become an HIV/AIDS self-manager and live your life better. This advice comes from physicians, health professionals, psychologists, and, most importantly, from people like you who have learned to manage living with their HIV/AIDS. Part 1 of the book, "HIV/AIDS Self-Management," will introduce you to the concepts and skills you need to become an HIV/AIDS self-manager. Part 2, "Managing Your Medical Treatment," discusses making treatment decisions. Part 3, "Managing Symptoms and Long-Term Health," will help you evaluate and begin to control some of the symptoms you may experience. Part 4, "Managing Exercise and Diet," contains information about healthy approaches to exercising and eating. And Part 5, "Managing Personal and Practical Issues," will help you approach some important issues of daily living and the losses caused by HIV/AIDS.

HIV/AIDS affects the lives of all kinds of people, with differing personal histories, sexual preferences, and cultural backgrounds. HIV/AIDS affects people who are HIV-positive without symptoms, in addition to those who develop symptoms or AIDS illnesses. And the people who *care about* people with HIV/AIDS and live with them and care for them—these people are also affected. This book will be helpful for all these people.

This is not a textbook—you don't have to sit down and read every word in every chapter. Instead, read the first two chapters and then use the table of contents to find what else you need. Many people pick and choose; feel free to skip around. You may want to start with some background information about HIV/AIDS and its symptoms and treatments. People who don't have symptoms may want to start by learning about exercise, healthy eating, and stress reduction. And people with all stages of HIV can use the knowledge here to help figure out whether a new symptom is a common "bug" or an urgent condition that needs to be checked out by the doctor. Become familiar with the information in the different parts, and use it in any order that's helpful for you.

This book is not a complete encyclopedia of HIV/AIDS. Information and resources for people with HIV/AIDS are always changing, so although we hope the leads given here will be useful, we intend them to be just good starting points. If you have good tips or helpful hints you want to pass on to others, please write us at the address below. We will incorporate them into future editions of this book.

Please send your ideas or tips to:

Allen L. Gifford, MD
University of California, San Diego
VA San Diego Healthcare System
3350 La Jolla Village Drive 111N-1
San Diego, CA 92161

PART ONE

HIV/AIDS
Self-Management

CHAPTER ONE

Overview of HIV/AIDS Self-Management

Times have changed. When we first started this book in the early 1990s, the dream of HIV/AIDS becoming a chronic illness was just that—a dream. Today many, if not most, people in treatment for HIV/AIDS live with the disease for many, many years. In fact, with treatment, HIV/AIDS has become a chronic condition similar to diabetes or heart disease. This is a very big step forward. Although we all celebrate this advance, it has brought with it a host of new questions: How do I balance my medication and my quality of life? Should I go on disability—which assures me of health care—or should I continue to work or go back to work? I look healthy—so to whom should I disclose that I have HIV/AIDS?

This book may not give you *all* the answers you seek, but it should give you many of the tools you need to deal with HIV and get on with your life. Let's start by discussing exactly what is meant when we talk about a chronic disease or condition. To do this it is important to know how acute and chronic diseases differ and why those differences matter.

ACUTE AND CHRONIC CONDITIONS

We think of a health problem as being either "acute" or "chronic." Acute health problems usually begin abruptly with a single, easily diagnosed cause;

they last for a limited time, and they often respond to a specific treatment, such as medication or surgery. Sometimes, as in the early day of AIDS, acute conditions end in death. For most acute illnesses, a cure with return to normal health is to be expected. For the patient and the doctor, there is relatively little uncertainty. One usually knows what to expect. The illness typically has a cycle of getting worse for a while, being treated, and then getting better. The care of an acute illness depends on a health profession-al's knowledge and experience to find and administer the correct treatment.

Appendicitis is an example of an acute illness. It typically begins rapid-ly, signaled by nausea and pain in the abdomen. The diagnosis of appen-dicitis, established by physical examination and lab tests, leads to surgery for removal of the inflamed appendix. There follows a period of recovery and then a return to normal health.

Chronic illnesses are different. They begin slowly and proceed slowly. For example, a person with arteriosclerosis ("hardening of the arteries") may have chest pains or breathing problems. Most arthritis starts with annoying little twinges, which gradually increase. Unlike acute disease, chronic illnesses often have many causes that vary over time and include heredity, lifestyle factors (smoking, lack of exercise, poor diet, stress, and so on), environmental factors, and physiological factors.

HIV/AIDS is a chronic disease and in many ways is quite similar to other chronic diseases, such as heart disease, stroke, and diabetes. Like these other diseases, HIV/AIDS is sometimes interrupted by acute infections or conditions. For example, a person with HIV may have day-in, day-out chronic symptoms of fatigue and then have a brief, acute episode of *Pneumocystis* pneumonia. Knowing the difference between the acute condi-tions and the chronic conditions associated with HIV/AIDS is quite impor-tant, because the acute conditions are sometimes infections (referred to as "opportunistic" infections) that need special treatment. Today, with increased use of medications, it is also important to know the difference between drug side effects and symptoms of HIV disease.

Chronic symptoms with multiple causes can be frustrating for those who want quick answers. It is difficult for the doctor and the patient when immediate answers aren't available. In some cases, even when diagnosis is rapid, as in the case of a stroke or heart attack, long-term effects may be hard to predict. Lack of a regular or predictable pattern is a major characteristic of most chronic illnesses—especially HIV/AIDS.

Unlike acute disease, in which full recovery is expected, chronic illness usually leads to persistent loss of physical conditioning. Because chronically ill people can tire easily, they may be unable to accomplish what they once could. They may give up recreational activities, such as walking or going to the gym, or chores like shopping, housework, and yard work. This lack of activity speeds up the process of physical deconditioning. At the same time, the loss of physical activity and uncertainty about the future can create a sense of helplessness, a feeling that little or nothing can be done to help the situation. Of course, believing that nothing can be done is a guarantee that nothing will be done, which reinforces helplessness and perpetuates the vicious cycle. A big problem in living with HIV/AIDS is dealing with this cycle of physical deconditioning (see Figure 1.1) and helplessness. Throughout this book we examine ways of breaking the cycle.

ACUTE VERSUS CHRONIC CONDITIONS		
Example	**Acute Condition** *Pneumocystis* pneumonia	**Chronic Condition** HIV/AIDS
Beginning	Rapid	Gradual
Duration	Short	Indefinite
Treatment	Cure common	Cure rare
Role of professional	Select and conduct therapy	Teach and advise
Role of patient	Follow professional's instructions/advice	Be active partner of health professionals, responsible for daily management

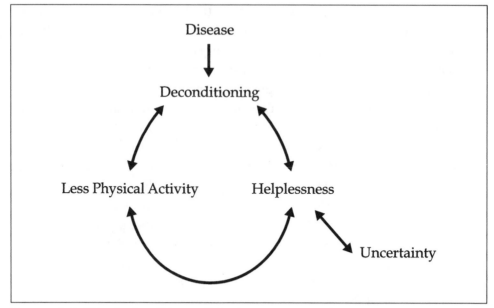

FIGURE 1.1 The Cycle of Deconditioning

Another way in which chronic illness differs from acute illness is that chronic illnesses such as heart disease, diabetes, and HIV/AIDS often have to be treated with medications that need to be taken every day, for life. Using medications properly is a big part of living with HIV/AIDS. We discuss medications at length in Chapter 6, "Managing Medications for HIV/AIDS," and Chapter 7, "Side Effects of Medications." Managing medications is just one part of self-management. Before discussing HIV/AIDS in more detail it is important to briefly discuss self-management.

HIV AND SELF-MANAGEMENT

For a person who has a disease like HIV/AIDS, it may seem overwhelming to think about being personally responsible for its management. Unfortunately, there is no alternative to self-management of a chronic condition. What are the options? One can go home and do nothing. This is a management style. One can decide to not take medications ordered by one's physician and instead to use alternative treatments. This too is a management style. One can decide to take a drug holiday. This is a management decision. In this book, we cannot tell you how to manage your HIV/AIDS. This is up to you. What we *can* do is give you all the information we have, including all the tools that others have found helpful in managing their HIV/AIDS. Using this knowledge, and the tools and advice you get from health professionals, family, and friends, you will make your own management decisions. There is no one best way—only the way that works best for you— but experience shows that active self-managers do better. The bottom line is that you want to run your disease, not let your disease run you. We will talk more about self-management later in this chapter and at length in Chapter 2, "Becoming an HIV/AIDS Self-Manager." Now let us examine exactly what HIV/AIDS is, and some of the associated conditions that accompany it.

UNDERSTANDING HIV AND AIDS

AIDS is a disease of the immune system caused by a virus—the human immunodeficiency virus, or HIV. People who become infected with HIV slowly develop damage to their immune systems. This usually takes months, or years. When the immune damage is minimal, a person with HIV doesn't notice anything at all. If the immune damage gets worse, the person may notice swollen lymph nodes or experience certain mild infections of the skin or mouth. If the immune damage gets quite severe, people with HIV lose the ability to fight off serious infections and cancers. If one or more of these serious infections or cancers develops, or if the immune system is very weak, the person is said to have AIDS: acquired immune deficiency syndrome.

In the next pages, we discuss how HIV is (and isn't) transmitted and what HIV does to the immune system. Some readers may find this information frightening, but it's impossible to be a self-manager without having knowledge of the basics. The reality is that most people today who are in treatment for HIV/AIDS can and do live fulfilling lives. As you learn the medical details about HIV/AIDS, it is important that you not lose track of three vital facts:

- HIV/AIDS is treatable. People in treatment who self-manage well can live long, healthy lives and feel better now than they ever could in the past.

- Treatments for HIV/AIDS are improving all the time. People starting treatment now have many more therapy options than ever before.

- Each person with HIV/AIDS has a unique experience. People can give you probabilities, but no one can say what will happen to you. For example, it's a mistake to assume that you will experience side effects from anti-HIV "cocktail" medication just because you know someone who did.

HOW DO PEOPLE CATCH AIDS?

Since AIDS is really the advanced form of infection with HIV, the real question is, "How do people catch HIV *infection?*" HIV infects only humans, and the only way it is transmitted is when the virus travels from inside one infected person to the bloodstream of another person. Some viruses, such as influenza (flu), concentrate in the lungs, so *coughing* spreads them around. Other viruses, such as chicken pox, concentrate in the skin, so *touching* an infected person can spread the disease. HIV is different. It concentrates in the blood and semen, and there aren't many ways to transfer blood and semen from one person to another.

Nearly all the known cases of HIV infection have been transmitted in one of the following ways:

- Sexual contact

- Injection with intravenous (IV) needles

- Transmission from a mother to her unborn child

- Transfusions of blood or blood products

Note that you can pass HIV on to someone else even while you are taking HIV medication, and even if your HIV viral load is very low, or undetectable. (You can read more about viral load tests in Chapter 5, "Making Treatment Decisions.") If you have ever been diagnosed with HIV you can always pass it on.

Sexual Contact

It is always risky for an HIV-positive person to have unprotected sex, but exactly how risky depends on what you do during sex. Unprotected anal sex is the most effective way to transmit HIV sexually. When a man with HIV puts his bare penis into another person's anus, the receiving person, whether a man or a woman, is at very high risk of catching HIV. Unprotected vaginal sex is also risky, although maybe a bit less risky than unprotected anal sex, since less cracking and bleeding of the skin occur.

There are two reasons why it is vital to practice safer sex if you are HIV positive:

- *To protect other people.* Obviously, you would not want to expose someone else to a serious illness.

- *To protect yourself.* Even if you are already HIV positive, you could be infected with new, possibly more dangerous strains of HIV. You could be infected with new HIV that is resistant to anti-HIV drugs. You will stay healthier longer if you can avoid any new HIV infection. If you have HIV, you are also at increased risk of getting other diseases like syphilis, gonorrhea, and hepatitis through unsafe sex because your immune system is compromised. And if you get one of these diseases your body will be less able to resist the infection and heal itself.

There are ways you can limit the risks to yourself and to others during sexual contact. Be aware of your body, and your partner's body. Cuts, sores, or bleeding gums increase the risk of spreading HIV. Even small injuries to the skin give HIV a way to enter the body. Use a barrier like a condom to prevent contact with blood or sexual fluid. The most common artificial barrier is the latex condom for men. You can also use a female condom to protect the vagina or rectum during intercourse. Lubricants can reduce the chance that condoms or other barriers will break. Oil-based lubricants like Vaseline, oils, or creams can damage condoms and other latex barriers; be sure to use water-based lubricants. Oral sex involves some risk of transmitting HIV, especially if sexual fluids enter the mouth and if there are bleeding gums or sores in the mouth. Pieces of latex or plastic wrap over the vagina, or condoms over the penis, can be used as barriers during oral sex.

Needles and Syringes

People who use a needle and syringe (the plastic container attached to the needle) to inject drugs leave a small amount of blood in the needle or syringe. If the needle or syringe is reused by someone else without being sterilized, the first person's blood will then be injected into the next person, causing transfer of the infection if the first person has HIV.

The best way to avoid HIV infection or transmission is to not use IV drugs. If you are injecting drugs, however, be sure to always use a new syringe and needle or clean the one you have. To do this, first fill the syringe to the top with clean water, shake it, and squirt it out three times. Repeat the procedure with 100% bleach, leaving the bleach in the syringe for at least 30 seconds each time you fill the syringe. Do this three times. Finally, fill the syringe with clean water, shake, and squirt the water out. Again, do this three times.

Mother to Child

The *placenta* is the organ inside a pregnant woman that allows food and oxygen from the mother to go to the unborn baby. If an HIV-positive woman is pregnant, the HIV in her blood can cross the barrier of the placenta and enter her baby's blood while the fetus is still in the womb. If the mother and the baby don't receive treatment, this kind of HIV transmission will happen in about one-third of babies born to HIV-positive women, and the baby will be born infected with HIV. BUT—and this is important—if women with HIV take medications while they are pregnant and the baby also gets medication at birth, this will block passage of HIV to the baby. *Thus if you are pregnant and have HIV, it is vital to get prenatal care as early as possible.* If you are pregnant and not sure about your HIV status, get tested as soon as possible. Be sure to tell your doctor what your HIV status is. Your baby's future health depends on you.

HIV can also pass from mother to baby in breast milk, although this means of transmission is much less common. In places like North America and Europe with access to safe alternatives to breast milk, most doctors recommend that women with HIV not breast-feed their babies. However, if baby formula and clean water are not available, breast milk may be the healthiest option for feeding your baby, even if you have HIV.

Blood Transfusion

Blood transfusions were an important source of HIV transmission until the blood test for HIV became available in 1985. Before 1985, blood banks couldn't tell which of the blood units they received had HIV and were therefore dangerous to give to others. Now the risk of getting HIV from a blood transfusion is extremely low.

Other Possible Ways to Catch AIDS

Everyone agrees how risky it is to have unprotected sex or to share dirty injection needles, but certain other activities are harder to be sure about. Kissing deeply with exchange of saliva is a good example of an activity people may have questions about. Saliva contains extremely low amounts of HIV, so infection from saliva is unlikely. Also, saliva has natural properties that limit the power of HIV to infect. But because of sores, bleeding gums, and bites, blood in the mouth is common and not always easy to detect. In theory, this blood could transmit HIV. In practice, no case of HIV infection has ever been proven to be caused by kissing.

WHAT DOES HIV INFECTION DO?

People who are infected with HIV experience a slow deterioration of their immune system. The immune system is vital to proper functioning of the human body, and that's why people with HIV infection can have so much trouble. The human immune system has many different components: There are infection-fighting white blood cells; there are messenger chemicals that signal parts of the system to turn on and off depending on what invader is causing problems; there are natural human toxins ("killer" chemicals) that can destroy invading organisms; and there are proteins that can "tag" invaders, making them more vulnerable to attack by the rest of the immune system. All parts of the immune system are important, but HIV attacks one part of the immune system in particular—a type of white blood cell known as the *T cell* (also called the *T helper, T4,* or *CD4+ cell*). People with HIV/AIDS have problems with specific types of infections and cancers that

WAYS OF CATCHING HIV FROM AN HIV-POSITIVE PERSON		
Definitely Risky	**Less Risky**	**Not Risky**
Unprotected anal sex	Mouth-to-genitals sex*	Shaking hands
Unprotected vaginal sex	Kissing with saliva exchange	Sharing bathroom
Sharing needles	Sharing razor or toothbrush	Touching doorknobs
Mouth-to-anus sex		Casual social contact
		Contact with sweat
		Insect bites

*Although unprotected oral sex is not as risky as anal or vaginal sex, research shows that it can transmit HIV.

are controlled by normal T cell function. You can read more about monitoring T cells in Chapter 5, "Making Treatment Decisions."

HIV can also infect brain cells, cells inside the bones (the bone marrow), and cells in the lining of the intestines. Because of the effect on brain cells, some people with advanced AIDS develop confusion and memory problems. Because blood cells are made in the bone marrow, the effect of HIV on the bone marrow can lead to decreased blood count (anemia). Chronic problems with diarrhea may come from the effect of HIV on the intestines.

It used to be that the average time from HIV infection to the development of full-blown AIDS was eleven years. This was an estimated average time for everyone with HIV, meaning that some people developed AIDS sooner and some later. Now we have stronger and better HIV medications, so people who take the medications can do very well even longer—for many years. No one can predict what will happen to any one individual.

HIV infection can be divided into four stages:

1. Primary HIV infection, or acute HIV

2. Healthy HIV carrier state

3. Early symptomatic HIV infection

4. AIDS

Primary HIV infection is the illness that occurs within two to four weeks after a person first has become infected with HIV. Not everyone has symptoms from primary HIV infection, but in some people it can cause fever, rash, sore throat, aching muscles, cough, swollen lymph nodes, diarrhea, nausea, and vomiting. In other words, it can be like a very bad flu infection. Primary HIV infection usually lasts only a few weeks, but many experts believe that seeing a doctor and having HIV detected during the primary infection is a big help. This may be a good time to start anti-HIV therapy. Unfortunately, though, most people don't have symptoms, or don't realize that the symptoms they get are from primary HIV.

After primary infection, a person with HIV goes into a healthy carrier state. During this phase, many people won't know that they have HIV, and they will feel fine—but unfortunately they still can transmit HIV to others.

People who develop symptomatic HIV infection will start to experience tiredness, fevers, skin and mouth infections, and abnormal blood tests. The immune system is weakened. If HIV infection continues untreated, the immune system becomes so weak that the person can develop serious infections and cancers—this stage is AIDS, the most advanced of the four stages.

When HIV infection becomes AIDS, the disease is serious, and can cause many symptoms. The line between having symptomatic HIV and having "full-blown AIDS" is not sharp. It's really a matter of degree of immune damage. Doctors use certain blood test measurements and refer to the presence of other infections in a person known to have HIV to define what they mean by "AIDS." Once people have AIDS, they have a lot of damage to their T cells and immune system. If they get a serious opportunistic infection like *Pneumocystis,* they're really sick. But remember, by using HIV medications and doing a good job self-managing their condition, even people who have AIDS can still rebuild their immune system and get healthy.

Health Problems and HIV

Most of the severe health problems that come from having HIV are caused by the infections and cancers that occur when the immune system gets weak. Because of effective medications for HIV, rates of AIDS-related infections and cancer have dropped sharply compared with fifteen years ago. The best way to prevent any of these illnesses is to use anti-HIV medications to boost the immune system. The most common HIV related illnesses are discussed in Chapter 3, "Health Problems of People with HIV/AIDS."

In addition to the problems directly associated with HIV/AIDS caused by a weakened immune system, people living with HIV have many of the same problems as they grow older that most other people face as they age. Living a full, long life with HIV is great, of course, but with aging can come symptoms from the heart, kidneys, liver, bones, and joints that often show up later in life. Because of this, many of the health problems of people currently living with HIV are chronic, and can come from aging, unhealthy habits, and side effects. Many people with HIV are prescribed multi-drug combinations of HIV medication, known as highly-active antiretroviral therapy (HAART) medications. (HAART refers to combinations of three or more strong anti-HIV drugs that are taken together.) Medications can lead to side effects. Even though the drugs can be lifesavers, a lot of chronic health care for people with HIV involves treating and managing those side effects. More and more people with HIV now have high cholesterol levels, high blood sugar, and increases in body fat. Because of drug side effects, and because people are living longer with HIV, they're also suffering from chronic heart disease, kidney disease, blood pressure, and liver problems just as many people do as they get older. There are also many problems and conditions that some people with HIV have that aren't actually *caused* by HIV—for example, excessive drinking and drug use, or depression. So when we talk about health problems with HIV, we really need to think about a lot of different things.

HIV/AIDS AS A CHRONIC DISEASE

HIV/AIDS can be similar to other chronic conditions in the sense that damage to the immune system may lead to problems with the lungs, causing the body to be deprived of oxygen, which leads to loss of function. But HIV can also lead to loss of function in other ways. Nerve cell damage caused by HIV can cause numbness or discomfort in the feet and hands. Problems in the intestines may decrease the absorption of fluids and important nutrients. Furthermore, the overall work that the body has to do to fight HIV in the cells can lead to an energy drain and fatigue. These things don't always happen, but if any one of them does, it can lead to pain and disability.

One does not always know that a chronic disease is present until the symptoms start (shortness of breath, fatigue, pain, and so on). Illness is more than cellular malfunction. It also includes problems with everyday life, such as not being able to do the things you want to do or needing to change your social activities, or needing to adapt life around the need for medications or tests.

Although the biological causes of chronic diseases differ, the problems they create are similar. For example, most people with chronic disease suffer fatigue and loss of energy. Sleeping problems are common. Some people may have pain, whereas others may have trouble breathing. Disability, to some extent, is also part of chronic disease.

Another common problem with HIV/AIDS and other chronic illnesses is depression, or just "feeling blue." It is hard to be cheerful when your condition causes serious health problems. Along with the depression come anger, fear, and concern for the future. Will I be able to remain independent? If I can't care for myself, who will care for me? What will happen to my family? Will I get worse? Will I be alone? What will happen as I age? Disability and depression bring loss of self-esteem. The management tasks and skills a person with HIV must learn are about the same for any chronic illness. Besides overcoming the physical and emotional problems, it is important to learn problem-solving skills and ways to respond to the trends in your disease. These tasks and skills include using medications appropriately and minimizing the side effects, developing and maintaining health with appropriate exercise and nutrition, managing symptoms, making decisions about when to seek medical help, working effectively with your doctor, finding and using community resources, talking about your illness with family and friends, and changing social interactions, if necessary. The most important skill of all is learning to respond to your illness on an ongoing basis to solve day-to-day problems as they arise.

In this book, we talk about learning to manage HIV/AIDS by applying the principles that have been successful in managing other chronic illnesses. Before we discuss specific management techniques, however, it is necessary to explain what we mean by self-management.

THE JOB OF SELF-MANAGEMENT

The first responsibility of any manager is to understand what is being managed. Initially, this may seem like an impossible task. After all, HIV/AIDS is a very complicated and challenging disease that sometimes stumps the best of specialists. But understanding HIV/AIDS is not as difficult as it might seem. Many people find that as a result of daily living with the consequences of the illness, they and their families become familiar with the way HIV affects them and what the treatment does for them. You will know better than anyone what problems you encounter with medications and side effects. With experience, you may become better able than health professionals to judge the course of your disease and the effects of your treatments. Most chronic illnesses go up and down in intensity; they do not have a steady path. Therefore, being able to identify the ups and downs in the path is essential for good management. These ups and downs can be important in making decisions about medications for pain, breathing problems, nausea, or other symptoms.

For example, the visits illustrated in Figure 1.2 represent Pat's regular follow-up appointments with the doctor. Even though the intensity of Pat's symptoms is the same for all three visits, what has happened between the appointments can make a big difference to the health care team in evaluating whether to change Pat's treatment or keep it the same. In the case of the January visit, the symptoms are getting better, so keeping the treatment the same or even lessening it may be in order. In the case of the February visit, the symptoms seem to be getting worse, so additional treatment may be the choice. In the case of the March visit, things have been stable for a while, so maintaining the treatment may be the best option.

Your experience and understanding of how you are doing are often a more useful indicator to your doctor than laboratory tests or other measures. If the physician encourages you to observe and to learn and you respond by participating in decisions, a partnership is born. To be most effective, self-management in HIV/AIDS requires such a partnership.

When you develop any chronic illness, you become more aware of your body. Minor symptoms that you used to ignore may now cause great concern. For example, is this cough a sign of pneumonia? Is this pain in my leg a sign that neuropathy (chronic nerve pain) has started? There are no simple, reassuring answers to apply to all patients. Nor is there a fail-safe way of sorting out serious signals from minor temporary symptoms that can be ignored. In general, symptoms should be checked out with your doctor.

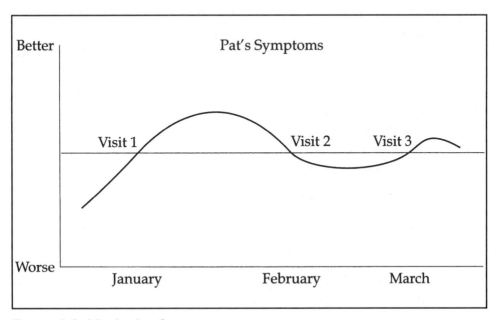

FIGURE 1.2 Monitoring Symptoms

This is especially true if the symptoms are unusual or severe, last more than a couple of weeks, or occur after starting a new medication. Some other guidelines about when to be concerned about symptoms are provided in Chapter 8, "Evaluating Common Symptoms of HIV/AIDS."

Throughout this book, we give specific examples of what actions to take if you experience certain symptoms. But since there is no "one size fits all" approach, this is where your partnership with your doctor becomes most critical. He or she can help guide you in responding to specific problems or symptoms. Self-management does not mean going it alone. Get help or advice when you are concerned or uncertain.

Both at home and in the business world, effective managers direct the show, but they don't do everything themselves. They work with others to get the job done. What makes them managers is that they are responsible for making decisions and making sure the decisions are carried out. As manager of your illness, your job is much the same. You gather information and work with a team of consultants consisting of your physician, other health professionals, and support people such as family and friends. Once they have given you their best advice, it is up to you to make decisions and follow through. All chronic illness needs day-to-day management. We have all noticed that some people with severe physical problems get on well, whereas other people with lesser problems seem to give up on life. The difference is often attitude and management style.

Managing a chronic illness, like managing a family or a business, is a complex undertaking. There are many twists, turns, and midcourse corrections. By learning self-management skills, you can ease the problems of living with your condition.

The keys to success in any undertaking are:

• Deciding what you want to do

• Deciding how you are going to do it

• Learning a set of skills and practicing until you have mastered them

These tasks are all based on learning skills and mastering them. Success in HIV/AIDS self-management is the same. In fact, mastering such skills is one of the most important tasks of life.

In this book, we describe several skills and strategies to help relieve the problems caused by HIV/AIDS. We do not expect you to use all of them. Pick and choose. Experiment. Set your own goals. What you do may not be as important as the sense of confidence and control you gain by successfully doing something that you want to do. However, we have learned that knowing the skills is not enough. You need a way of incorporating them into your daily life. In trying a new skill, the first attempts are usually clumsy and slow and show few results. It is easier to return to old ways than to continue trying to master new and sometimes difficult tasks. The best way to master new skills is through continued practice and evaluation of the results.

SELF-MANAGEMENT SKILLS

What you do about something is largely determined by how you think about it. For example, if you think that having HIV is like running in the dark toward a cliff, not knowing when you will fall over the edge, you might feel no control over what happens and therefore do nothing at all to help yourself. The thoughts you have can greatly determine what happens to you and how you handle your health problems.

The most successful self-managers are people who think of their illness as a path rather than as a cliff. This path, like any path, goes up and down. Sometimes it is flat and smooth. At other times the way is rough. To negotiate this path you have to use many strategies. Sometimes you can go fast; at other times you must slow down. Effective self-managers are people who have learned the skills to negotiate this path.

Self-management skills fall into three main categories:

- *Skills needed to deal with the illness.* Any illness requires that you do new things. These may include taking many medicines and sticking to complicated medication schedules. Sometimes there are new exercises or a new eating plan. Taking care of the illness also means more frequent interaction with your doctor and the health care system. All of these constitute the work you must do to manage your illness.

- *Skills needed to continue your normal life.* Just because you have HIV does not mean that life stops. There are still chores to do, friendships to maintain, jobs to do, and many family relationships to carry on. Things that you once took for granted can become much more complicated in the face of HIV/AIDS. You may need to learn new skills in order to maintain your daily activities and to enjoy life.

- *Skills needed to deal with emotions.* When you are diagnosed as having HIV/AIDS, your future changes, and with this come changes in plans and emotions. Many of these emotions are negative. They may include anger ("Why me? It's not fair"), depression ("I can't do anything anymore. What's the use?"), frustration ("No matter what I do, it doesn't make any difference. I can't do what I want to do"), or isolation ("No one understands. No one wants to be around someone who is sick"). Negotiating the path of HIV, then, also means learning skills to work with negative emotions.

In the next chapter, we discuss more about what it means to be a self-manager and how you can master the skills necessary to be one. Throughout the book you will find information to use as you go about the important task of becoming a successful HIV/AIDS self-manager.

SELF-MANAGEMENT TASKS

- *Taking care of your illness* (taking medicine, exercising, going to the doctor, changing diet)

- *Carrying out your normal activities* (household chores, employment, social life, and so on)

- *Managing your emotional changes* (working with changes brought about by your illness, such as anger, uncertainty about the future, altered expectations and goals, and sometimes depression. Changes can also occur in your relationships with family and friends.)

CHAPTER TWO

Becoming an HIV/AIDS Self-Manager

Like any skill, self-management must be learned and practiced. This chapter will start you on your way. Remember, *you are the manager*. Like the manager of an organization or household, you must have a management plan:

1. *Decide* what you want to accomplish.

2. *Look for alternative ways* to accomplish this goal.

3. Start making short-term plans by *making an action plan* or agreement with yourself.

4. *Carry out your action plan.*

5. *Check the results.*

6. *Make changes* as needed.

7. Remember to *reward yourself.*

Problems sometimes start with a general uneasiness. You are unhappy but not sure why. Upon closer examination, you find you miss contact with old friends who live far away. With the problem identified, you decide to take a trip to visit your friends. You know what you want to accomplish. In the past, you could have easily driven, but you now find it tiring, so you seek alternative plans for travel. Among other things, you consider leaving at noon instead of early in the morning, and making the trip in two days instead of one. You consider asking a friend along to share the driving. There is also a train that goes within twenty miles of your destination, or you might fly (although this is more expensive). You decide to take the train. The trip still seems overwhelming, as there is so much to do to pre-pare. You decide to write down all the steps necessary to make the trip a reality. These include finding a good time to go, buying a ticket, figuring out how to handle luggage, and thinking about how you can manage your medications and meals when you're away from home.

You start by making an action plan or agreement with yourself that this week you will call and find out just how much the railroad can help. You also decide to review your medication schedule and meal plans to make sure you have what you need for the trip. You then carry out your action plan by calling the railroad and checking your medication and meal needs.

A week later, you check the results. Looking back at all the steps to be accomplished, you find that a single call answered many questions. The rail-road is able to accommodate your needs for special meals. However, you are still worried about storing your medications during the trip. You make a change in your plan by asking a friend about this, and he suggests a place where you can buy special travel containers for all your medications.

Now you are ready to make a new action plan for accomplishing some of the other tasks necessary to make the trip possible. What once seemed like a dream is becoming a reality.

Let's go through these seven steps in detail. They are the backbone of any self-management program.

DECIDING WHAT YOU WANT TO ACCOMPLISH

Deciding what you want to accomplish may be the most difficult part. You must be realistic and very specific. Think of all the things you would like to do. One of our self-managers wanted to climb twenty steps to his friend's home so he could join his friend's family for a holiday meal. Another want-ed to gain weight to improve his strength. Still another wanted to be more socially active even though he felt limited by the need to take an oxygen tank everywhere. In each case, the goal was one that would take several weeks or even months to accomplish. In fact, one of the problems with goals is that they often seem like dreams. They are so far off that we don't even try to accomplish them. We'll tackle this problem next. For now, take a moment to write your goals below. When you have finished, put an asterisk (*) next to the goal you would like to work on first.

GOALS

1. _____

2. _____

3. _____

LOOKING FOR ALTERNATIVE WAYS OF ACCOMPLISHING THE GOAL

Sometimes what keeps us from reaching our goal is a failure to see alternatives. Other times, we reject alternatives without knowing much about them.

There are many ways to reach any specific goal. For example, our self-manager who wanted to climb twenty steps could start off with a slow walking program, start to climb a few steps each day, or look into having the family gathering at a more accessible location. The man who wanted to gain weight could decide to keep a log of his daily calorie intake, talk to his doctor about changing some of his medications, or start an exercise program. The self-manager who wanted more social contact could find out about community college classes or support groups, or could call or write friends.

As you can see, there are many options for reaching each goal. The job here is to list the options and then choose one or two on which you would like to work. Sometimes it is hard to think of all the options yourself. If you are having problems, it is time to use a consultant. Share your goal with family, friends, and health professionals. You can call community organizations such as your local AIDS Foundation or Project Inform. (These are just two of many community and national organizations available to people with HIV/AIDS and their friends and families. There's more information about these resources in Chapter 17, "Finding Resources.") Rather than ask what you should do, ask for suggestions. It is always good to have a list of options.

Sometimes people don't consider an option because they assume it doesn't exist or is not workable. Try not to make this kind of assumption without investigating first. One woman we know had lived in the same town all her life and felt that she knew all about the community resources. When she was having problems with her health insurance, a friend from another city suggested contacting an insurance counselor. The woman dismissed this suggestion, however, because she knew that this service did not exist in her town. Months later the friend came to visit, called the area social service agencies (listed in the telephone book), and located three insurance counseling services. In short, never assume anything. Assumptions are the major enemies of the self-manager.

Once you have identified your options, write them on the following lines and put an asterisk (*) next to the two or three options on which you would like to work first.

OPTIONS

1. _____

2. _____

3. _____

4. _____

5. _____

6. _____

MAKING SHORT-TERM PLANS: ACTION PLANNING

The next step is to turn your options into a short-term plan, which we will call an action plan. An action plan calls for a specific action or set of actions that you can realistically expect to accomplish within the next week. The action plan should be about something you want to do or accomplish. You do not make action plans to please your friends, family, or doctor, but rather to please yourself.

Most of us can do things to make ourselves healthier, but we fail to do them. For example, most people with HIV/AIDS can walk—some just across the room, others for a mile, others much farther. However, few people adhere to a systematic exercise program. An action plan helps you do the things you know you should do and want to do. Knowing how to make a realistic action plan is an important skill that may well determine the success of your self-management program.

1. First, *decide what you will do* this week. For the step-climber mentioned earlier, this might be climbing three steps every day for four days. The man trying to gain weight may decide to eat six small meals per day. The action must be something you want to do and realistically feel you can do—a step on the way to your long-term goal. Make sure that your plans call for a *specific* action or behavior; that is, rather than just saying you will "relax," decide that you will "listen to the progressive muscle relaxation tapes."

2. Next, *make a specific plan*. This is the most difficult and important part of making an action plan. Deciding what you want to do is worthless without a plan for doing it. The plan should contain all of the following parts:

   • Exactly *what* are you going to do? How far will you walk, how will you eat better, what breathing technique will you practice?

   • *How much* will you do? Will you walk around the block, eat at least two fruits per day, practice breathing exercises for fifteen minutes?

   • *When* will you do the activity? Again, this must be specific: before lunch, in the shower, when you come home from work? Connecting a new activity (walking) with an old habit (taking a lunch break) is a good way to make sure it gets done. Another trick is to schedule your new activity before an old favorite activity, such as reading the paper or watching a favorite TV program.

- *How often* will you do the activity? This is a bit tricky. We would all like to do things every day. However, because we are human, this is not always possible. It is usually best to plan to do something three or four times a week. If you do more, so much the better. **Please note:** Taking medications is an exception. Medicine must be taken exactly as you and your doctor have agreed. Otherwise you will never know whether the medications help, and you may put yourself and others in great danger.

Here are a couple of guidelines for writing your action plan that may help you achieve success:

- *Start where you are, or start slowly.* If you can walk for only one minute, start your walking program by walking one minute once every hour or two, not by trying to walk a mile. If you have never done any exercise, start with a few minutes' warm-up. A total of five or ten minutes is enough. If you want to lose weight, set a goal based on changing your eating behaviors, such as not eating after dinner.
- *Give yourself some time off* (again with the exception of taking medication). All people have days when they don't feel like doing anything. It is better to say you will do something three times a week instead of every day. That way, if you don't feel like walking one day, you can still meet your action plan.

Once you've made your action plan, ask yourself the following question: "On a scale of 0 to 10, with 0 being totally unsure and 10 being totally sure or confident, how confident am I that I can complete this action plan?"

If your answer is 7 or above, yours is probably a realistic action plan. Congratulate yourself—you have done the hard work. If your answer is less than 7, then you should look at your plan again. Ask yourself why you're not

> ### QUALITIES OF AN ACTION PLAN
>
> 1. Something *you* want to do
>
> 2. Reasonable (something you can expect to do this week)
>
> 3. Behavior specific
>
> 4. Answers the questions: What? How much? When? (Think about your day and week—which days, which times?) How often?
>
> 5. Confidence level of 7 or more (that you will complete the entire action plan)

confident. What problems do you foresee? Then see if you can either solve the problems or change your plan to make yourself more confident of success.

Once you have made an action plan you are happy with, write it down and post it where you will see it every day. Keep track of how you are doing and what problems you encounter. We've included an example of an action plan form at the end of this chapter. You may want to make copies of it to use weekly.

CARRYING OUT YOUR ACTION PLAN

If your action plan is well thought out and realistic, fulfilling it is generally pretty easy. Ask family or friends to check with you on how you are doing. Having to report your progress is good motivation.

Keep track of your daily activities while carrying out your plan. All good managers have lists of what they want to accomplish. Check things off as they are completed. This will give you guidance on how realistic your planning was, and it will also be useful in making future plans. Make daily notes, even of the things you don't understand at the time. Later these notes may help you to see patterns and to solve problems.

For example, our stair-climbing friend had trouble getting around to his climbing practice. Each day he encountered a different problem: not enough time, being tired, bad weather, and so on. When he looked back at his notes, he began to realize that the real problem was his fear of getting short of breath and falling. So he modified his plan: He decided to do strengthening and breathing exercises, and to climb the stairs when a friend or neighbor was around.

CHECKING THE RESULTS

At the end of each week, see if you have completed your action plan and if you are any nearer to accomplishing your goal. Are you able to walk farther? Have you gained weight? Are you less fatigued? Taking stock is important. You may not see progress day by day, but you should see a little progress each week. At the end of each week, check on how well you have fulfilled your action plan. If you are having problems, this is the time to problem-solve.

MAKING MIDCOURSE CHANGES: PROBLEM SOLVING

When you are tying to overcome obstacles, your first plan may not always be the most practical one. If something doesn't work, don't give up. Try something else: Modify your short-term plans so that your steps are easier, give yourself more time to accomplish difficult tasks, choose new steps to your goal, or check with your consultants for advice and assistance.

1. The first and most important step is to *identify the problem*. This is usually the most difficult step as well. You may know, for example, that keeping up with your work and social activities is a problem for you, but it will take a little more effort to determine that the real problems interfering with your activities are managing medications and fatigue.

2. Once you have identified the problem, the next step is to *list ideas to solve the problem*. You may be able to come up with a good list yourself, but calling in help from consultants is often beneficial. Consultants may be friends, family, members of your health care team, or community resources.

3. When you have a list of ideas, *pick one to try.* As you try something new, remember that new activities are usually difficult. Be sure to give your potential solution a fair chance before deciding it won't work.

4. After you've given your idea a fair trial, *assess the results.* Was the idea helpful? If all has gone well, your problem will be solved.

5. If you still have the problem, *choose another idea* from your list and try again.

6. If a solution still eludes you, *use other resources* (your consultants) to get more ideas.

7. If none of the above steps works, you may have to *accept that your problem may not be solvable right now.* This is sometimes hard to do. However, just because a problem is not solvable right now doesn't mean that it won't be solvable later or that other problems can't be solved with this method. Even if your path is blocked, there may be alternative paths. Don't give up. Keep going.

PROBLEM-SOLVING STEPS

1. Identify the problem. (This is the most difficult and most important step.)

2. List ideas to solve the problem.

3. Select one method to try.

4. Assess the results.

5. Substitute another idea if the first one doesn't work.

6. Utilize other resources (ask friends, family, and professionals for ideas if your solutions don't work).

7. Accept that the problem may not be solvable now.

REWARDING YOURSELF

The best part of being a good self-manager is the rewards you will receive by accomplishing your goals and living a fuller and more comfortable life. However, don't wait until your ultimate goal is reached—reward yourself frequently. For example, decide that you won't read the paper until after you exercise. Reading the paper then becomes your reward. One self-manager rewards himself with an ice cream cone after finishing each of his medical appointments. Another self-manager who stopped smoking used the money he would have spent on cigarettes to have his house professionally cleaned; there was even enough left over to go to a baseball game with a friend! Rewards don't have to be fancy, expensive, or unhealthy. There are many healthy pleasures that can add enjoyment to your life.

One last note: Not all goals are achievable. Chronic illness may mean having to give up some options. If this is true for you, don't dwell too much on what you can't do. Rather, start working on another goal you would like to accomplish. One self-manager we know who uses a wheelchair talks about the ninety percent of things he *can* do. He spends his life developing this ninety percent to the fullest.

THE SUCCESSFUL SELF-MANAGER

- Sets goals
- Makes a list of alternatives for reaching a goal
- Makes short-term plans or action plans toward that goal
- Carries out the action plan
- Checks on progress weekly
- Makes midcourse changes as necessary
- Uses rewards for a job well done

ACTION PLAN FORM

In writing your action plan, be sure it includes

- What you are going to do

- How much you are going to do

- When you are going to do it

- How many days a week you are going to do it

For example: This week, I will walk (*what*) around the block (*how much*) before lunch (*when*) three times (*how many*).

This week I will:

_____ (*what*)

_____ (*how much*)

_____ (*when*)

_____ (*how many*)

How confident are you that you can complete this action plan?

_____

(Write a number between 0 and 10, where 0 = not at all confident and 10 = totally confident)

	Check Off	Comments
Monday	_____	_____
Tuesday	_____	_____
Wednesday	_____	_____
Thursday	_____	_____
Friday	_____	_____
Saturday	_____	_____
Sunday	_____	_____

Now that you understand the meaning of self-management, you are ready to begin using the tools that will make you a self-manager. In Chapters 3 through 7, we talk about HIV-related health problems, treatment, and medications. Chapters 8 and 9 contain information on some of the common chronic symptoms with HIV. The rest of the book is devoted to self-management skills. These include exercise, nutrition, symptom-management, communication, making decisions about the future, finding resources, and information about advance directives. You do not have to read things in order. Skip around. As a self-manager, how you use this book is up to you.

CHAPTER THREE

Health Problems of People with HIV/AIDS

Good HIV self-management is only possible with a basic knowledge of some key facts about HIV, including an understanding of the health problems that people with HIV can develop. Many people living with HIV infection feel fine, and of course that's exactly the goal of good anti-HIV treatment. However, if and when people do get sick, they may have problems that come from the HIV infection itself, or they may have problems related to side effects of medicines they take. They may also get sick as a result of the health risks that people with HIV often take, habits they may have, or due to aging itself. Whatever the cause, good self-management skills will help the person with HIV figure out the best strategy for dealing with these health problems. In this chapter we look briefly at some of the health problems most often seen in those with HIV.

MEDICAL PROBLEMS CAUSED BY UNCONTROLLED HIV INFECTION

With the advent of effective medications for HIV, rates of these AIDS infections, cancers, and nerve problems have dropped sharply. However, when HIV is not controlled and the immune system gets weak, people can suffer from numerous illnesses and get infections and cancers that are very serious. Uncontrolled HIV can also harm the brain and nerves, causing people to have memory problems and pain. You may have heard of some of the following illnesses referred to as *opportunistic infections.* "Opportunistic infection" is a general term for the serious infections that people with HIV can get if the immune system becomes weak. The best way to prevent these illnesses is to use medications to control HIV and boost the immune system.

Pneumocystis jiroveci (Formerly *Pneumocystis carinii*) Pneumonia (PCP)

Pneumocystis jirveci is a new name for the parasite that used to be called *Pneumocystis carinii*—but it's really the same type of HIV-related pneumonia (lung infection) that was once the most common AIDS-related illness in the United States. In fact, since they are the same, even though the formal name has changed, we still refer to *Pneumocystis* as PCP—not PJP—when we abbreviate the name. We're now much better at preventing *Pneumocystis* with anti-HIV and anti-*Pneumocystis* medicines, but PCP is still one of the more common and most serious AIDS illnesses. People at high risk for PCP can often avoid getting the disease by taking low doses of PCP drugs such as trimethoprim/sulfamethoxazole (i.e., Bactrim, Septra) daily.

Bacterial Pneumonia

Pneumonias caused by common bacteria are an important problem for people with HIV. These bacterial pneumonias can be treated with antibiotics if they're caught early, and vaccines can help prevent them from ever occurring. The flu vaccine helps, too, since the flu virus can lead to bacterial pneumonia. Medicines to prevent PCP (such as Septra or Bactrim) can also help to prevent bacterial infection. Part of good self-management is to be sure you receive a vaccination for pneumonia—this is usually done every five years—and be sure you get an annual flu shot.

Candida

Candida, also called thrush, is a fungus that is commonly found in the mouth, skin, gastrointestinal tract, and vagina. Candida takes the form of white spots or patches that can be easily scraped off with a stick. Candida of the esophagus (the swallowing tube between the mouth and stomach) is a common AIDS illness in the United States and is serious because it makes it painful to swallow and thus interferes with eating. Candida of the vagina can be quite mild but it is also sometimes painful. For some people, candida is the first sign of problems with the immune system. Antifungal medicines are usually very effective.

Kaposi's Sarcoma (KS)

Kaposi's sarcoma is a type of slow-growing skin cancer that initially appears as a purple, brown, or pink bump on the skin. It may be very limited and not cause much trouble, but sometimes it can spread widely on the skin and even to the internal organs. Kaposi's sarcoma is seen mostly in gay men; it is rare in heterosexuals and even in IV drug users. When it's mild, KS may not require any treatment at all. But in severe cases, anticancer drugs (chemotherapy) or other treatments may be necessary.

HIV Wasting Syndrome

People with HIV/AIDS can lose weight because of the direct effects of the virus on their bodies, and also because they have problems with eating and absorbing food. Wasting is often associated with fevers. Once weight is lost, it may be very difficult to regain. Losing more than 10% of body weight (that is, 15 pounds in a 150-pound person) is a sign of HIV wasting syndrome, and losing as little as 5% of body weight is significant.

It is important to treat wasting syndrome quickly, because advanced wasting can be very dangerous. People with wasting also have a big problem with lack of energy. Your doctor will want to make sure there is no treatable infection other than HIV that's causing problems with your stomach or intestines. A regimen of effective HAART (Highly-Active Antiretroviral Therapy) drugs is often the best way to treat wasting, so it can be important to start, or to adjust these. High-calorie food supplements and drinks can help, as can special medications to stimulate the appetite or boost the body hormones that help store calories.

Toxoplasmosis of the Brain

Toxoplasmosis, also called "toxo," is caused by a parasite (*Toxoplasma gondii*) found in undercooked meat; it is a common infection in humans and many animals. *Toxoplasma* is also often found in cat litter boxes, soil, and other places where animals leave their waste. Because of this, people with HIV/AIDS need to be careful to wear gloves when changing cat litter or working in the garden. In healthy people, toxo causes very few problems; for most people, the immune system controls the infection without any trouble. In people with HIV, however, the infection can move to the brain and cause weakness, seizures, or problems with speech or walking. It can travel to the internal organs as well. Toxo can be prevented by taking trimethoprim/sulfamethoxazole. If toxo is contracted but is caught early enough, toxoplasmosis can be controlled by taking medicines such as pyrimethamine and sulfadiazine.

Mycobacterium avium Complex (MAC) or *Mycobacterium avium intracellular* (MAI)

Mycobacterium avium is a kind of bacteria that can spread widely through the blood and internal organs of people with advanced HIV/AIDS. Usually, MAC is seen when the T cell count has dropped below 100. People who have a blood CD4+ cell count of less than 50 cells per microliter should take an antibiotic such as azithromycin regularly to *prevent* MAC. Once the infection starts, treating MAC is more difficult; it usually requires taking two or three different types of antibiotics for long periods, perhaps indefinitely.

Cytomegalovirus (CMV)

Cytomegalovirus is a very common virus that most people have been exposed to long before they ever become infected with HIV. Only when the immune system is weakened does CMV start to cause problems in the eyes, the intestinal tract, and sometimes other internal organs. The virus can damage the back of the eye (CMV retinitis), causing partial loss of vision and even blindness in severe cases. In the intestinal tract (CMV colitis or enteritis), CMV causes pain, ulcers, bleeding, and diarrhea. Like MAC, CMV is usually seen when the T cell count has dropped below 100.

Medication can slow and sometimes even stop the problems caused by CMV. The medications can be given orally, or through an intravenous line (IV) in the arm or chest. Boosting T cells with HIV medications may also slow or stop the effects of CMV disease.

Tuberculosis (TB)

Tuberculosis is one of the most common and serious infections throughout the world. It can be found in non-HIV-infected people as well as in those with HIV, but people with HIV contract TB much more easily and in a more severe form. Tuberculosis is caused by *Mycobacterium tuberculosis,* a bacterium that infects mostly the lungs, although it can spread throughout the body in some people with AIDS.

Tuberculosis is particularly common in people who lack good access to medical care. It causes cough, fever, and weight loss and spreads easily through the air around a person coughing out the TB bacteria. Fortunately, many people who have been exposed to TB can be identified through skin tests. People on effective TB treatment can no longer pass the disease to others. Treatment for TB may call for four or more oral medicines, which usually must be given for a year or more. Staying on the TB medicine is very important—not only for the well-being of the person with TB, but also to protect others from getting the disease.

Herpes Infections

There are two main types of herpes viruses: herpes simplex and herpes zoster. Herpes simplex type I causes sores (commonly known as cold sores) mostly on the mouth and lips; herpes simplex type II causes sores on the genitals and anus. Sometimes herpes simplex can spread to other parts of the body. Herpes zoster is caused by varicella, the same virus that causes chicken pox. It often leads to *shingles,* a painful rash that appears on one section of the skin. In severe cases, herpes zoster can spread to other parts of the body. If the infection spreads to the eyes, it can endanger the vision. Either type of herpes can affect people who don't have HIV, but for people with HIV, herpes is often one of the early infections they experience. Medicines are available to treat herpes simplex infections, but herpes zoster and other types of herpes are quite difficult to treat.

Cryptosporidiosis

In cryptosporidiosis, a parasite (*Cryptosporidium parvum*) infects the intestines and can cause diarrhea and stomach cramps. The parasite is found in many animals and is passed on when food or water is contaminated. People with normal immune systems get rid of the parasite quite easily; those with weakened immune systems may never do so. Unfortunately, cryptosporidiosis is very difficult to treat. It is important that people with this disease avoid getting too dehydrated, and that they strengthen their immune systems and boost T cells by taking combination HIV medications.

Lymphoma

Lymphoma is a cancer of the lymph system caused by uncontrolled growth of abnormal white blood cells. The most common lymphoma in people with HIV is a type called non-Hodgkin's lymphoma. Symptoms include fever or night sweats with painless enlargement of a lymph node (gland) in only one part of the body. It also can start in the brain and cause headaches, localized weakness, speech problems, or seizures. Non-Hodgkin's lymphoma is very difficult to treat.

Cervical Pathology (Abnormal Pap Smear)

Women with HIV often have abnormal changes in their cervix (the neck and opening of the womb). Doctors sometimes call this condition "dysplasia" or "atypia." Without careful monitoring and treatment, the condition can develop into cancer of the cervix. If you are a woman with HIV, it's important to have regular pelvic examinations to be sure that if a problem develops, you can detect it and take care of it early, before it spreads. If you smoke, it's a good idea to quit, since smoking seems to increase the risk of cervical cancer.

Dementia

Problems with memory and slowed-down thinking may result from HIV disease. If the disease is advanced and levels of HIV in the blood are high, HIV dementia can be more of a problem. However, because almost everyone forgets things sometimes, it really takes a doctor to figure out whether a person may be experiencing HIV dementia. For people who do have dementia, it's important to have a support system. Friends and partners can help with things like remembering when to take HIV medications each day. Lots of people keep cues around them (such as notes, calendars, or alarms) to remind themselves about medicines, appointments, and other important things. Treatment with HIV medications may help control dementia by reducing the HIV that enters the brain.

Neuropathy

Pain or tingling in the feet or hands can be caused by peripheral neuropathy, a nerve problem caused by HIV disease. Neuropathy can be very uncomfortable for some people, sometimes making it hard to function. Treatment depends on the exact cause of the problem: Some people will improve if they adjust their HIV medications, others may need to use pain medications. Many people with neuropathy benefit from taking other medications that affect the nerves, such as depression or seizure medications.

OTHER HEALTH PROBLEMS OF PEOPLE WITH HIV

Of course, people with HIV also have health problems not directly caused by the virus or their weakened immune systems. In fact, the more HIV treatments improve, the more we need to think about the *other* health problems people have. Conditions that people with HIV often have, but that aren't directly caused by HIV, are called *comorbidities*. Here are a few of the most common ones.

Hepatitis C Virus (HCV)

Hepatitis C virus is an infection of the liver that is common in people with HIV because, like HIV, it can be spread via needles and sex. People with HCV may not have symptoms from it for many years, but eventually they can have damage to the liver and, later, complete liver failure. It is very important that people with HCV not do things that damage the liver, like drink alcohol (beer, wine, or other liquor). It's also important to have regular liver tests. HCV can be treated and sometimes even cured with medications such as pegylated interferon alfa and ribavirin. But these drugs aren't easy to take—they can cause side effects like body aches and depression. Still, with support from your medical team, taking the drugs to treat HCV can be worth it.

Depression

Many people with HIV experience serious depression, with reduced quality of life and faster progression of HIV disease. Sometimes there is a real risk of suicide. People with depression may have trouble eating or sleeping, and they may feel tired all the time, or worthless and guilty. Be very careful about drugs and alcohol—they may seem like ways to cheer up, but in people with depression they just make matters worse and can be dangerous. Depression can be treated, but many people don't talk to their doctors about it, and the doctors may not ask. If you think you are depressed, you must let your doctor know. If you start on an antidepressant medication, expect it to take two to four weeks before you notice any improvement. For more discussion of HIV and depression, see Chapter 9, "Understanding the Symptom Cycle."

Changes in Fat and Metabolism

People using HAART (Highly-Active Antiretroviral Therapy) medications to treat their HIV may experience changes in the way fat is distributed on their bodies. This is called *lipodystrophy*. (For many people, this is a big issue, so we discuss it in detail in the next paragraph.) Some people also experience changes in their cholesterol levels and blood sugar. These changes are worrisome because they may increase the risk of heart disease or strokes. Because these changes are due mostly to drug side effects, we also discuss them in Chapter 7, "Side Effects of Medications."

Lipodystrophy, or change in body shape, is a common complication of HIV/AIDS. It was first thought to be a side effect of taking protease inhibitors. However, lipodystrophy sometimes occurs in people who are not taking these drugs, and occasionally even in people with HIV who have never used HAART drugs. Whatever the cause, lipodystrophy can be very annoying and sometimes frightening. Fat moves from the legs and buttocks to the abdomen, breasts, and neck. These changes can be accompanied by

changes in cholesterol and blood sugar, so they should not
Treatment may include changing drugs, exercise, and surgical
the fat. Experimental approaches, including use of a drug based
growth hormone, are also being tried. Please see Chapter 11, "Exercising
for Fun and Fitness," for more information about how exercise can help
this condition.

Given the host of potential health problems for people with HIV, you
can see that it is vitally important to carefully manage your medical treatments. The chapters that follow in Part 2, "Managing Your Medical
Treatment," provide vital information on the roles and uses of medications,
how to work with your doctor, and how to make treatment decisions.

SUGGESTED READING

Bartlett, John G., and Finkbeiner, Ann K. *The Guide to Living with HIV
Infection: Developed at the Johns Hopkins AIDS Clinic.* 5th ed. Baltimore,
Md.: The Johns Hopkins University Press, 2001.

PART TWO

Managing Your Medical Treatment

CHAPTER FOUR

Working with Your Doctor

With all the new tests, medications, and research coming out, it might seem that HIV care is impossibly complicated, and that patients should just go to the doctor, listen, and do as the doctor says. However, that's not the way chronic diseases work. Patients with chronic diseases spend very little time with their health care providers. They act as their own "first-line" caregivers—taking medications on their own, and monitoring their daily activities and symptoms on their own or with family members. No matter how complicated or technical your HIV treatment is, no one knows better than you what problems are arising on a day-to-day basis and how the care plan fits into your routine.

People with chronic HIV take care of themselves, but the help of their doctors, nurses, and other experts is critical to doing that. So to live well with HIV you need to be able to work with your doctor; that means being able to choose a doctor and to talk with him or her about your treatments and about how you're doing, and about what you should do. These are the topics we will discuss in this chapter.

CHOOSING A DOCTOR

Finding the right doctor is a concern for most people, and even more so for a person with HIV. There are many different kinds of doctors out there, and sometimes it is difficult to know which type of doctor is right for you.

Although you may need to work with a specialist at times for specific problems, no one type of specialty training is always necessary for treating HIV/AIDS. But it is best to find a doctor who is familiar with the needs of people with HIV and who can help you with all of your health care. Usually, this is an internist for adults and a pediatrician for children.

An internist has had special training in the care of adults and can care for most common adult health problems. A pediatrician has had special training in the care of children. Not all internists, pediatricians, or even different specialists, however, are experienced in treating HIV/AIDS. For this reason, when choosing your doctor, look for one who has this experience, preferably one who has many HIV patients as part of his or her practice. Many doctors with HIV experience have special training in infectious diseases, but this is not mandatory to be an excellent HIV doctor.

Another factor to consider when choosing your doctor is that he or she be someone you like, and can get along with. The sooner you can find such a doctor, the sooner you can begin to build a partnership and develop the best treatment plan for your condition. Being able to establish and maintain this relationship, though, means learning effective ways to communicate with your doctor, especially given the time constraints you must work with during your visits.

COMMUNICATING WITH YOUR DOCTOR

The relationship you have with your doctor must be looked on as a long-term one requiring regular work, much like a close partnership. Your doctor will probably know more intimate details about you than anyone except perhaps your spouse, partner, or parents. You, in turn, should feel comfortable expressing your fears, asking questions that you may think are "stupid," and negotiating a treatment plan to satisfy both you and your doctor without feeling "put down" or ignored.

In this partnership between you and your doctor, the biggest threat to a good relationship and good communication is lack of time. If you or your doctor were to fantasize about the best thing to happen in your relationship, it would probably involve more time for you both—more time to discuss things, more time to explain things, more time to explore options. When time is short, the resulting anxiety can lead to rushed communication—messages that may be misunderstood—and there is no time to correct miscommunication.

A doctor is usually on a very tight schedule. This fact becomes painfully obvious when you have to wait in the doctor's office because an emergency has come up. Doctors try to stay on schedule, and sometimes patients and doctors alike feel rushed as a consequence. One way to help you get the most from your visit with the doctor is to take **PART**—*P*repare, *A*sk, *R*epeat, *T*ake action.

Prepare

Before visiting or calling your doctor, prepare your "agenda." What are the reasons for your visit? What do you expect from your doctor? Take some time to make a written list of your concerns or questions. But be realistic. If you have thirteen different problems, it isn't likely that your doctor can adequately deal with that many concerns in one visit. Identify your *main* concerns or problems. Writing them down helps you remember them. Have you ever thought to yourself, after you walked out of the doctor's office, "Why didn't I ask about. . . ?" or "I forgot to mention. . . ." Making a list beforehand helps to ensure that your main concerns get addressed.

Preparing will also help you do several important things *during* the visit.

- *Mention your main concerns right at the beginning of the visit.* Give your list to the doctor, and let him or her know which items are the most important to you. If the list is long, expect only two or three items to be addressed in this visit. Studies show that doctors allow an average of eighteen seconds for the patient to state his or her concerns before interrupting with focused questioning. Preparing your questions in advance will help you use your eighteen seconds well. Remember to check your list before you leave to make sure your most important concerns have been addressed.

Here's an example of how to bring up your major concerns at the beginning of the visit. When the doctor asks, "What brings you in today?" you might say something like "I have a lot of things I want to discuss this visit." (*The doctor immediately begins to feel anxious because of an already overfilled appointment schedule.*) "But I know that we have a limited amount of time. The things that most concern me are my dizziness and the side effects from one of the medications I'm taking." (*The doctor feels relieved because the concerns are focused and potentially manageable within the appointment time.*)

- *Describe your symptoms concisely.* This includes when they started; how long they last; where they are located; what makes them better or worse; whether you have had similar problems before; whether you have changed your diet, exercise, or medications in ways that may contribute to the symptoms; and so on. If a treatment has been tried, you should be prepared to report the effect of the treatment. And if you have previous records or test results that may be relevant to your problems, bring them along.

- *Be as open as you can in sharing your thoughts, feelings, and fears.* Remember, your physician is not a mind reader. If you are worried, try to explain why: "I am afraid that what I have may be contagious" or "I'm worried the virus has become resistant." The more open you are, the more likely it is that your doctor can help you.

- *Give your doctor feedback.* If you don't like the way you have been treated by the doctor or someone else on the health care team, let your doctor know. If you were unable to follow the doctor's advice or had problems with a treatment, tell the doctor so that adjustments can be made. Also, most doctors appreciate compliments, but patients are often hesitant to praise their doctors. If you are pleased, remember to let the doctor know this, too.

Ask

Another key to effective doctor-patient communication is asking questions. Getting understandable answers and information is one of the cornerstones of self-management.

You need to be prepared to ask questions about diagnosis, tests, treatments, and follow-up.

- *Diagnosis.* Ask your doctor what's wrong, what caused it, whether it's contagious, what the future outlook (or prognosis) is, and what can be done to prevent it in the future.

- *Tests.* Ask your doctor if more medical tests are necessary, how they will affect your treatment, how accurate they are, and what is likely to happen if you are not tested. If you decide to have a test, find out how to prepare for the test and what it will be like.

- *Treatments.* Ask about your treatment options, including different kinds of medication options. Inquire about the risks and benefits of treatment and the consequences of not treating.

- *Follow-up.* Find out if and when you should call or return for a follow-up visit. What symptoms should you watch for, and what should you do if they occur?

You may want to take some notes during the visit or consider bringing along someone to act as a second listener. Another set of eyes and ears may help you remember details of the visit or instructions later.

Repeat

It is extremely helpful to briefly repeat back to the doctor some of the key points from the visit and discussion, such as diagnosis, prognosis, next steps, and treatment actions. This allows you to double-check that you clearly understood the most important information. It also gives the doctor a chance to quickly correct any misunderstandings and miscommunications. If you don't understand or remember something the physician said, admit that you need to go over it again. For example, you might say, "I'm pretty sure you told me some of this before, but I'm still confused about it." Don't be afraid to ask what you may think is a "stupid" question. Such questions can often bring out an important concern or clear up a misunderstanding.

Take Action

When the visit is ending, make sure you clearly understand what to do next. When appropriate, ask your physician to write down instructions or recommend reading material for more information on a particular subject.

If, for some reason, you can't or won't follow the doctor's advice, let the doctor know. Be honest, even if you're worried that what you're saying isn't what the doctor wants to hear. For example, "I can't take the Viracept. It gives me stomach problems, and I always miss the dose in the middle of the day," or "My insurance doesn't cover that, so I can't afford it," or "I've tried to quit smoking before, but everyone I know smokes, and I just can't stay off cigarettes." If your doctor knows why you can't or won't follow the advice, he or she can sometimes make suggestions to help you overcome the barrier. If you aren't open about the barriers to taking action, it's difficult for your doctor to help.

TALKING TO YOUR DOCTOR ABOUT MEDICATIONS

It is common for people with HIV to be taking lots of medications: anti-HIV HAART (highly-active antiretroviral therapy) medications, anti-inflammatory drugs for pain or fever, a pill for depression, an antibiotic pill to prevent *Pneumocystis,* antacids for heartburn, a tranquilizer for anxiety, plus a handful of over-the-counter (OTC) remedies. *Remember, the more medications you are taking, the greater the risk of drug side effects.* Fortunately, you can often reduce the number of medications and the associated risks if you have forged an effective partnership with your doctor. Such a relationship requires your participation in determining the need for the medication, selecting the medication, properly using the medication, and reporting back to your doctor the effects of the medication.

An individual's response to a particular medication varies depending upon age, metabolism, activity level, and the waxing and waning of symptoms caused by most HIV diseases. Many medications are prescribed on an as-needed (PRN) basis, so you need to know when to begin and end treatment and how much medication to take. You need to work out a plan with your doctor to suit your individual needs.

For most medications, *your doctor depends on you* to report what effect, if any, the drug has on your symptoms and what side effects you may be experiencing. On the basis of that information, your doctor may continue, increase, discontinue, or otherwise change your medications. A good doctor-patient partnership requires a continuing flow of information. There are important things you need to let your doctor know and critical information you need to receive in return.

Unfortunately, this vital interchange is too often shortchanged. Studies indicate that fewer than five percent of patients receiving new prescriptions ask any questions of their physicians or pharmacists. Doctors tend to interpret patient silence as understanding and satisfaction with the information received. Mishaps often occur because patients either do not receive adequate information about medications and don't understand how to take them, or fail to follow instructions given to them. Safe, effective drug use depends on your understanding of the proper use, the risks, and the necessary precautions associated with each medication you take. *You must ask questions.*

The goal of treatment is to maximize the benefits and minimize the risks. Whether the medications you take are helpful or harmful often depends on how much you know about your medications and how well you communicate with your doctor.

What You Need to Tell Your Doctor

Even if your doctor doesn't ask, there is certain vital information you should mention to him or her.

Are you taking any medications?

Report to your physician and dentist *all* the prescription and nonprescription medications you are taking, including experimental medicines, herbs, birth control pills, vitamins, aspirin, antacids, and laxatives. This information is especially important if you are seeing more than one physician because one may not know what the others have prescribed. Knowing all the medications you are taking is essential for correct diagnosis and treatment. For example, symptoms such as nausea, diarrhea, sleeplessness, drowsiness, dizziness, memory loss, impotence, and fatigue may be due to a drug side effect rather than a disease.

It is critical for your doctor to know what medications you are taking to help prevent problems from drug interactions. Carry an up-to-date list with you, or at least know the names and dosages of all the medications you are taking. Saying that you are taking "the little green pills" usually doesn't help identify the medication. Everyone should get into the habit of doing a "brown bag" medicine check at least once every six months. The idea is simple: Put all the medicines you're taking into a bag, and bring them with you when you see your doctor. Review *all* the medicines with your doctor, and make sure you know which to continue and which to stop or discard. Don't forget the over-the-counter and the "as-needed" medications!

Have you had allergic or unusual reactions to any medications?

Describe any symptoms or unusual reactions to medication you have taken in the past. Be specific: Which medication and exactly what type of reaction? A rash, fever, or wheezing that develops after you take a medication is often a true allergic reaction. If any of these symptoms develops, call your doctor at once. Nausea, ringing in the ears, lightheadedness, and agitation are likely to be side effects rather than signs of true drug allergies.

Do you have any major chronic diseases or medical conditions other than HIV?

Many diseases can interfere with the action of a drug or increase the risk of using certain medications. Diseases involving the kidneys or liver are especially important to mention, because these diseases can slow the metabolism of many drugs and increase toxic effects. Your doctor may also have you avoid certain medications if you have or have had such diseases as hypertension, peptic ulcer disease, asthma, heart disease, diabetes, or prostate problems. Be sure to let your doctor know if you could be pregnant or are breast-feeding, since many drugs are not safe to use in those situations.

What medications were tried in the past to treat your disease?

If you have a chronic symptom or symptoms, it is a good idea to keep your own written record of what medications you have taken for the condition and what the effects were. Knowing your past responses to various medications will help guide the doctor's recommendation of any new medications. However, just because a medication did not work well in the past does not necessarily mean that it shouldn't be tried again today or in the future. Diseases change and may become more responsive to treatment.

What You Need to Ask Your Doctor

Do I really need this medication?

Some physicians decide to prescribe medications not because they are really necessary, but because they think patients want and expect drugs. Don't pressure your physician for medications. If your doctor doesn't prescribe a medication, consider that good news rather than a sign of rejection or indifference. Ask about non-drug alternatives. Many conditions can be treated in a variety of ways, and your physician can explain your options. In some cases, lifestyle changes such as exercise, diet, and stress management should be considered before other choices. When any treatment is recommended, ask what the likely consequences are if you postpone treatment. Sometimes the best medicine is none at all.

What is the name of the medication?

If a medication is prescribed, it is important that you know its name. Write down both the brand name and the generic (chemical) name. If the medication you get from the pharmacy doesn't have the same name as the one your doctor prescribed, ask the pharmacist to explain the difference.

What is the medication supposed to do?

Your doctor should tell you why the medication is being prescribed and how it is expected to help you. Is the medication intended to prolong your life, completely or partially relieve your symptoms, or improve your ability to function? For example, if you are given an anti-HIV drug such as AZT (Retrovir), the purpose is primarily to prevent or slow deterioration of your immune system. It probably won't stop all of your HIV-related symptoms, and it may have side effects. On the other hand, if you are given a skin cream, the purpose is to help ease your skin condition.

You should also know how soon you should expect results from the medication. Drugs that treat infections or inflammation may take several days to a week to show improvement, whereas antidepressant medications typically take several weeks to begin working.

How and when do I take the medication, and for how long?

Understanding how much of the medication to take and how often to take it is critical. Does "every 6 hours" mean "every 6 hours while awake"? Should the medication be taken before meals, with meals, or between meals? What should you do if you accidentally miss a dose? Should you skip it, take a double dose next time, or take it as soon as you remember? Should you continue taking the medication until the symptoms go away or until the medication is completely used up?

The answers to such questions are very important. For example, if you are taking an antibiotic for a lung infection, you may feel better within a few days, but you should continue taking the medication as prescribed to completely eliminate the infection; otherwise, the infection may come back, perhaps in a stronger, drug-resistant form. Didanosine (ddI, Videx) must be taken two pills at a time and chewed or crushed in order to be effective. If you are using an inhaled medication for breathing problems, the way you use the inhaler determines how much of the medication actually gets into your lungs. Taking medication properly is vital. Yet when patients are surveyed, nearly forty percent report that they were not told by their physicians how to take the medication or how much to take. If you are not sure about your prescription, call your doctor or nurse. Such calls are never considered a bother.

What foods, drinks, other medications, or activities should I avoid while taking this medication?

Having food in your stomach may help protect the stomach from some medications, whereas it may render other drugs ineffective. For example, milk products or antacids can decrease the absorption of some drugs (such as Nizoral) but may increase the absorption of others (such as Fortovase). Some medications may make you more sensitive to the sun, putting you at increased risk for sunburn. Ask whether the medication prescribed will interfere with driving. Other drugs you may be taking, even OTC drugs and alcohol, can either amplify or lessen the effects of the prescribed medication. The more medications you are taking, the greater the chances of undesirable drug interactions. So ask about possible drug-drug and drug-food interactions.

What are the most common side effects, and what should I do if they occur?

All medications have side effects. You need to know what symptoms to be on the lookout for and what action to take if they develop. Should you seek immediate medical care, discontinue the medication, or call your doctor? Your doctor cannot be expected to list every possible adverse reaction, but the more common and important ones should be discussed. Unfortunately, a recent survey showed that seventy percent of patients starting a new medication did not recall being told by their physicians or pharmacists about precautions and possible side effects. So it may be up to you to ask.

Are tests necessary to monitor the use of this medication?

Some medications are monitored by the improvement or worsening of symptoms. However, many medications used to treat people with HIV can disrupt body chemistry before any telltale symptoms develop. Sometimes these adverse reactions can be detected by laboratory tests such as blood counts or liver function tests. In addition, the level of some medications in the blood need to be measured periodically to make sure you are getting the right amount. Ask your doctor if the medication being prescribed has any of these special requirements.

Can a generic medication that is less expensive be prescribed?

Every drug has at least two names, a generic name and a brand name. The generic name is the nonproprietary, or chemical, name of the drug. The brand name is the manufacturer's unique name for the drug. When a drug company develops a new drug in the United States, it is granted exclusive rights to produce that drug for seventeen years. After the seventeen-year period has expired, other companies may market chemical equivalents of that drug. These generic medications are generally considered as safe and effective as the original brand-name drug but often cost half as much. Because many HAART drugs are quite new, often no generic equivalent is available. Right now, there are no generic anti-HIV HAART medications in the United States (though some generics are available in other countries).

Even so, if cost is a concern, ask your doctor if there is a lower-cost but equally effective medication. Sometimes you can save money by purchasing medications through the mail. Many health maintenance organizations (HMOs) and mail-order pharmacies offer prescription services.

Is there any written information about the medication?

Realistically, your doctor may not have time to answer all of your questions in detail. Even if your physician carefully answers your questions, it can be difficult for anyone to remember all this information. Fortunately, there are many other valuable sources you can turn to: pharmacists, nurses, package inserts, pamphlets, books, and the Internet. Some particularly useful sources to consult are listed in the "Suggested Resources" section at the end of Chapter 6, "Managing Medications for HIV/AIDS."

A SPECIAL WORD ABOUT PHARMACISTS

Your pharmacist is an expert on medications. You can often call him or her on the phone to find out about medications and how they work. In addition, many hospitals, medical schools, and schools of pharmacy have medication information services you can call to ask questions. As a self-manager, don't forget pharmacists. They are important and helpful consultants.

SUGGESTED READING

Jones, J. Alfred, Kreps, Gary L., and Phillips, Gerald M. *Communicating with Your Doctor: Getting the Most out of Health Care.* Creskill, N.J.: Hampton Press, 1995.

CHAPTER FIVE

Making Treatment Decisions

HIV treatment has changed dramatically during the last few years. There are now many more medications available to help people with HIV. While this is good, it has also made the decisions about what medications to take and when to start treatment more difficult. In this chapter we discuss some important aspects of monitoring HIV as well as self-management and how it applies to making decisions about medications and other treatment options.

MONITORING HIV AND YOUR IMMUNE SYSTEM

People with HIV may get lots of different blood tests, but two blood tests are particularly important for monitoring HIV and helping you and your doctor to make treatment decisions. The first is the viral load test, also called the HIV plasma RNA test or the PCR test. The second is the T cell or CD4+ cell test. It is important that you know the basics of these tests to understand and consider treatments for HIV.

HIV Viral Load Test

The HIV virus is constantly multiplying in a person with HIV, but whether it multiplies quickly or slowly depends on the immune system and on the medications being used. Measuring the level of HIV in the blood is a way of telling how active the virus is. The more HIV in the blood, the more quickly the virus can damage the immune system. People with a high level of HIV activity in their blood (high viral load) and more immune system damage are generally advised to take anti-HIV medications like HAART (highly-active antiretroviral therapy). People with very low HIV activity in their blood (low viral load) and less immune system damage may be advised to wait.

There are different tests to measure HIV in the blood, but they all count the number of HIV particles (HIV RNA) in the blood. Measurements are usually reported as the number of virus copies in each milliliter of blood. The virus may be undetectable (usually fewer than 50 copies), it may be detectable but low (fewer than 10,000–30,000 copies per milliliter), or it may be quite high (over a million copies). Because the numbers range so widely, a tenfold or even a hundredfold drop in viral levels is possible with effective treatment. This means that someone with 100,000 HIV copies per milliliter before treatment could drop to 1000 copies per milliliter with effective treatment.

T Cell or CD4+ Cell Count

Whereas the viral load test tells how active the virus is, the T cell count is the best test for monitoring how much HIV has affected the immune system, and how strong the immune system is. The T cell count is simply a blood test that measures the number of T helper cells (or CD4+ cells) in each microliter of blood. Because T cells are important in fighting infections and cancers, having a low T cell count increases the risk of illness. But T cell counts change quite a bit, even in healthy, HIV-negative people. All kinds of things affect the T cell count, such as stress, sleep, time of day, the lab where the test was done, and whether the patient has other infections. The T cell count is a bit like your blood pressure: It's important, but it goes up and down, and the overall trend is more important than any one reading.

Generally speaking, a T cell count between 500 and 1800 is normal for adults. A count between 200 and 500 indicates that the immune system is weakened, but people in this range are usually not at high risk of getting seriously ill. AIDS diseases usually don't affect people with a T cell count over 200. Kaposi's sarcoma (KS), tuberculosis (TB), and lymphoma are exceptions, but when a person's T cell count is over 200, these diseases are less dangerous. Problems like oral candida (thrush) and skin problems can also appear when the T cell count is over 200.

A T cell count between 50 and 200 indicates that the immune system is severely weakened. One of the ways doctors decide who has HIV that is severe enough to be AIDS is to ascertain whether the T cell count is 200 or less. Many opportunistic infections (infections that develop when the immune system is weak but not when it's strong) occur when the T cell count is 200 or lower. People with T counts lower than 200 definitely should take medication to prevent *Pneumocystis* pneumonia (PCP). Even though they need to take medication, lots of people with T cells lower than 200 may feel healthy and have no symptoms.

A T cell count below 50 indicates that the T cell part of the immune system is not functioning. Good, comprehensive medical care is vital, and treatment with medicines to prevent opportunistic infections is very important. Most people who die of AIDS have a T cell count below 50. However, even at this low count, some people will feel well and have no AIDS-related problems. So T cells are important, but they're not the whole story.

Both the HIV load and the T cell count must be considered in order to monitor how an individual person is doing. Of course, it's always best to have a high T cell count and a low (or undetectable) viral load. But people with low T cell counts can still do quite well if the viral load is also low, indicating that no further weakening of the immune system is taking place. Researchers have developed charts that show how likely it is that a person with HIV will become sick with AIDS, based on their viral load and T cell count. This kind of information is important when making decisions about medications.

STARTING ANTI-HIV THERAPY

Nearly everyone who is getting care for HIV or AIDS knows about *Highly Active AntiRetroviral Therapy—HAART*, the "cocktail" combinations of medications used to treat HIV. One of the most important things that you need to be able to discuss with your doctor is when to start taking HAART. The decision to start taking HAART is not simple. It's especially difficult if you feel well and have no symptoms from HIV. However we know that high levels of HIV in the blood will make people sick eventually, so it makes sense to take medication to lower the viral load.

The HIV medications now available are very good. They perform miracles for some people. But at the same time, taking medications is work. It requires effort to remember to take the pills, to follow all the instructions for taking them properly, to deal with any side effects or inconveniences that the medications cause, and to fit the medications into your daily routine. So in a way, the short answer to the question of when to start taking anti-HIV drugs is this: Start on the drugs when you *want* to, and when you *can*. Of course, figuring this out isn't easy. Each person with HIV has to work on this with his or her doctor.

As you think about your decision, you and your doctor will want to consider both medical issues, related to the immune system and the virus, and personal issues, related to your own strengths and priorities. To decide when to start, it will help to consider the recommendations compiled by experts. The accompanying table, "Making the Decision to Start on HAART," is based on recommendations from the Panel on Clinical Practices for Treatment of HIV Infection, convened by the U.S. Department of Health and Human Services and the Henry J. Kaiser Family Foundation. If you have HIV and you've never been on anti-HIV medications, take a look at the table and bring it in to discuss with your doctor. It will be a good starting point for weighing the risks and benefits of treatment.

General recommendations don't always fit every individual. Here are some of the questions you'll need to talk through with your doctor:

- How much is your immune system already affected? What is the CD4+ or T cell count?

- How much risk is there that the disease will progress? What is the viral load (plasma HIV RNA level) now?

- How motivated are you to start the medications?

- After you've gotten all the help possible from your health care team, friends, and family, how confident are you that you can take the anti-HIV medications exactly as they're supposed to be taken?

MAKING THE DECISION TO START ON HAART

Symptoms	T Cell Count and HIV Viral Load	Recommendation
No symptoms	T cell count greater than 350 cells per microliter and HIV viral load lower than 100,000 copies per milliliter	Do not start HAART. Simply watch and wait.
No symptoms	T cell count greater than 350 cells per microliter and HIV viral load greater than 100,000 copies per milliliter	Most experts recommend simply watching and and waiting. Some, however, may recommend that you consider HAART.
No symptoms	T cell count between 201 and 350 cells per microliter	HAART should be seriously considered.
No symptoms	T cell count lower than 200 cells per microliter	HAART is recommended.
Any AIDS-defining illness oral thrush, fevers, or other severe HIV symptoms	Any value	Treatment is recommended.

Adapted from the Panel on Clinical Practices for Treatment of HIV Infection, U.S. Department of Health and Human Services and the Henry J. Kaiser Family Foundation.

- Are the potential benefits of starting the medications greater than the risks?

Working out the answers to these questions may not be easy or straight-forward. You may want to get the opinion of a second doctor, or talk with people who are already using the medications. Thinking about these issues and discussing them is really necessary so that you can make an informed decision.

OTHER HIV-RELATED TREATMENTS TO KEEP YOU HEALTHY

The anti-HIV HAART medications are important, but they're certainly not the *only* important part of medical care for a person with HIV. Much of the trouble people with HIV have is caused by the opportunistic infections and cancers we discussed in Chapter 3, "Health Problems of People with HIV/AIDS." So in addition to taking your HAART medications, use other strategies to help prevent disease:

- Strengthen your immune system against infections by keeping current with immunizations.

- Eliminate traces of infection with preventive antibiotics, before the infection develops into disease.

- Detect signs of infection early, so it can be treated before causing prob-lems.

- Change your lifestyle to promote or maintain general good health.

To make sure you're getting the best care possible, you must stay up-to-date on basic prevention strategies. The tables on the next few pages list the basic tests, medications, and vaccines recommended for adults with HIV/AIDS (children are different—don't use these guidelines for them). Remember, these are basic guidelines; you and your doctor may decide to do things differently, depending on your circumstances. But if you decide *not* to do one of the things listed, it should be because you've thought about it, talked to your doctor about it, and made an informed and careful decision. That's the essence of being a self-manager.

To use the tables, look under the correct heading for your T cell count and make sure that you and your doctor do each of the things listed. Prepare by making a list to bring to the doctor's office.

WHEN YOU BEGIN CARE FOR HIV (ANY T CELL COUNT) . . .

Get These Tests

Plasma HIV RNA concentration (HIV viral load)

T-cell count (CD4+ and CD8+ cells)

Complete blood count (white blood cells, anemia, platelets)

Complete blood chemistry profile, including liver enzyme tests

Fasting blood glucose and blood cholesterol tests

Baseline syphilis blood test

Baseline hepatitis A, B, and C blood tests

Toxoplasmosis antibody test

Urinalysis test

Consider and discuss HIV resistance testing

Baseline chest X-ray

Baseline electrocardiogram (if over age 40)

Baseline vaginal and pelvic exam, and Pap test (women)

Baseline oral/dental exam

Baseline physical exam

Skin test for tuberculosis (PPD* tuberculin test)

Skin test for anergy**

* Purified protein derivative.

** Anergy skin testing verifies that your immune system can respond to skin tests.

CONTINUED ON NEXT PAGE

WHEN YOU BEGIN CARE FOR HIV (ANY T CELL COUNT) . . .

Get These Vaccines
Diptheria-tetanus (every 10 years)
Pneumococcal vaccine (every 10 years)
Influenza vaccine (every fall/winter)
Hepatitis A vaccine (if hepatitis A blood test is
negative)
Hepatitis B vaccine (if hepatitis B blood test is
negative) (a single series of three shots)

Make a Decision
Evaluate your symptoms, viral load, and T cell
count, and *discuss anti-HIV medications with
your doctor* (see "Starting Anti-HIV Therapy,"
page 59).

About Medications
If your PPD test is positive and X-ray shows no
active TB, take recommended medication for
one year to prevent TB.

Be a Self-Manager
Find a health care provider who you like and
can talk to, and who knows about HIV. Think
hard about changing your health habits—
practicing safer sex and getting off drugs,
smoking, and alcohol.

*   Purified protein derivative.
** Anergy skin testing verifies that your immune system can respond to skin tests.

IF YOUR T CELL COUNT IS GREATER THAN 200 . . .

Get These Tests
Plasma HIV RNA concentration (HIV viral load) every 3–6 months
CD4+ T cell count every 3–6 months
Syphilis blood test every year, or after new sexual exposure
Prompt exam by eye doctor if vision problems develop
Vaginal and pelvic exam, and Pap test (women) every 6–12 months
Oral/dental exam every 6 months
Routine physical exam every 6 months
Skin tests for tuberculosis (PPD tuberculin test) and anergy every 6 months

Get These Vaccines
Influenza vaccine (every fall/winter)

Make a Decision
Evaluate your symptoms, viral load, and T cell count and

About Medications
Discuss anti-HIV medications with your doctor (see "Starting Anti-HIV Therapy," page 59). If your PPD test is positive and X-ray shows no active TB, take recommended medication for one year to prevent TB.

Be a Self-Manager
Educate yourself about HIV and the medications available.
Build a strong partnership with your doctor.
Think hard about changing your health habits —practicing safer sex and getting off drugs, smoking, and alcohol.

If Your T Cell Count Is Less than 200 . . .

Get These Tests
Plasma HIV RNA concentration (HIV viral load) every 3–6 months

CD4+ T cell count every 3–6 months

Syphilis blood test every year, or after new sexual exposure

Prompt exam by eye doctor if vision problems develop

Vaginal and pelvic exam, and Pap test (women) every 6–12 months

Oral/dental exam every 6 months

Routine physical exam every 6 months

Skin tests for tuberculosis (PPD tuberculin test) and anergy every 6 months

Get These Vaccines
Influenza vaccine (every fall/winter)

Make a Decision
Evaluate your symptoms, viral load, and T cell count and

About Medications
Discuss starting HAART medications with your doctor (see "Starting Anti-HIV Therapy," page 59).

Take TMP/SMZ,* dapsone, or inhaled pentamidine to prevent *Pneumocystis* pneumonia.

If your T cell count is lower than 100 cells/μl, take TMP/SMZ* or dapsone-pyrimethamine to prevent toxoplasmosis.

If your T cell count is lower than 50 cells/μl, take recommended medication to prevent *Mycobacterium avium* complex (MAC).

CONTINUED ON NEXT PAGE

IF YOUR T CELL COUNT IS LESS THAN 200 . . .	
	If your PPD test is positive and X-ray shows no active TB, take recommended medication for one year to prevent TB.
Be a Self-Manager	Educate yourself about HIV and the medications available.
	Build a strong partnership with your doctor.
	Make sure you know about your doctor's night/weekend coverage system, in case you need it.
	Exercise and eat nutritious foods.
	Think hard about changing your health habits—practicing safer sex and getting off drugs, smoking, and alcohol.

* Trimethoprim/sulfamethoxazole.

SUGGESTED READING

AIDS Treatment News. ATN, Philadelphia FIGHT, 1233 Locust St., 5th Floor, Philadelphia, PA 19107. (A semi-monthly newsletter reporting on HIV/AIDS treatments.) Published by John S. James. (800-TREAT-1-2)

Bartlett, John G., and Finkbeiner, Ann K. *The Guide to Living with HIV Infection,* developed at The Johns Hopkins AIDS Clinic. 5th ed. Baltimore, Md.: The Johns Hopkins University Press, 2001.

Grodeck, Brett. *The First Year—HIV: An Essential Guide for the Newly Diagnosed.* New York: Marlowe, 2003.

CHAPTER SIX

Managing Medications for HIV/AIDS

Having HIV/AIDS usually means taking medications. Therefore, a very important self-management task is to understand your medications and use them appropriately. In this chapter we discuss general issues relating to the role of medications in fighting HIV/AIDS, and specific medications that may be prescribed to you, including highly-active antiretroviral therapy (HAART) drugs and preventive and treatment medications. Our goal in this chapter is to arm you with some of the basic information you'll need to effectively self-manage your medications for HIV. HIV treatment is complicated. Even experienced doctors and other health care workers need all their professional skills and knowledge to do it well. But a person with HIV needs to know the basics, too.

A Few General Words about Medications and HIV

Almost nothing is as aggressively advertised as medications. When we read a magazine, listen to the radio, log onto e-mail, or watch TV, we are bombarded with a constant stream of ads aimed at convincing us that if we just take this pill or that tablet, our symptoms will be cured. "Recommended by ninety percent of doctors surveyed!" "Shouldn't *you* try Zocor?" Almost as a backlash to this advertising, we have been taught to avoid excess medications. We have all heard about or experienced some of the ill effects of medications. The media also tell us, "Just say 'no' to drugs" and "Drugs can kill." It is all very confusing.

Even so, medications are a very important part of managing HIV/AIDS. So far, medications cannot completely cure the disease, but they can do many things to help people live well:

- Medications that fight HIV directly (such as HAART medications) can reduce the level of virus and *slow or stop the disease process*. For example, drug combinations such as indinavir (Crixivan), lamivudine (3TC, Epivir), and zidovudine (AZT, Retrovir) can reduce the effects of HIV and improve the immune system.

- Medications can help *prevent problems from starting*. For example, people at high risk for *Pneumocystis* pneumonia can take medicines to keep from ever getting the disease. In pregnant women with HIV, HAART medications can prevent the baby in the womb from getting HIV/AIDS.

- Medications can *reduce symptoms* through their chemical actions. For example, pain medications decrease activity in nerve cells, which can decrease pain sensations. Nausea medications decrease stomach hyperactivity, which relieves stomach upset.

- Finally, there are medications that *replace substances that the body is no longer producing adequately*. Hormones such as testosterone and epoetin (Procrit) are medications of this type.

In all cases, the purpose of medication is to lessen the consequences of disease or to slow its course. However, many of the drugs doctors prescribe will not have an immediate positive effect that you can feel instantly when you take them. Sometimes a drug will stabilize a condition that would have gotten worse without the drug. Sometimes a drug may only slow down a deterioration that would have been more rapid without the drug. It can be easy to think that the drug isn't doing anything. Except for drugs that are taken just for symptoms, it's hard to judge just by how you feel whether medications are working. This is why it's important to talk openly with your doctor about your medications and discuss any changes you may want to make. This is especially true with anti-HIV HAART medications. If you stop taking some of them, or if you skip doses, you may make the HIV in your body resistant, so that your HIV gets stronger rather than weaker and the disease gets worse instead of better.

WHAT MEDICATIONS ARE AVAILABLE TO TREAT HIV/AIDS?

The main treatments used for HIV/AIDS are medications that act in one of four ways:

- *Antivirals* (or *antiretrovirals*) fight the HIV itself by preventing the virus inside the body from reproducing. Protease inhibitors, reverse-transcriptase inhibitors, fusion inhibitors, and all the other HAART drugs work this way.

- *Preventive medicines* prevent specific opportunistic infections. People with HIV are carefully monitored to find out when they are at high risk for certain specific diseases. Then, if they move into a high-risk group, they can start taking preventive medicines. Preventive strategies for *Pneumocystis*, tuberculosis, toxoplasmosis, and *Mycobacterium avium* complex (MAC) are effective and well established.

- *Treatment medicines* are used to treat specific opportunistic infections and diseases once they are identified.

- *Immune boosters* are taken to increase the body's immune response to invaders and to HIV itself. This approach may be promising for the future, but presently it is still experimental and there are no approved treatments of this type. The therapeutic vaccines that are being developed are in this category. Some researchers think that immune boosters will someday be necessary if we hope to completely cure people with HIV.

In this chapter we discuss some of the more common medications used in HIV care. However, new medications for HIV/AIDS are being developed all the time, and much more extensive and detailed descriptions of older and newer HIV medications are widely available in books or on the Internet[1] (see "Suggested Reading" at the end of this chapter).

USING ANTIVIRAL (HAART) MEDICATIONS

Many different types of medications are prescribed for people with HIV, including antibiotics that fight a variety of infections, and medications that treat symptoms such as pain and depression. But anti-HIV (antiviral or anti-retroviral) drugs are the ones that specifically attack HIV itself. These drugs are the main treatment for HIV, and improvement in these types of drugs in recent years has made a dramatic difference in many people's lives.

HAART antiretroviral medications get the most attention of the medications used by people with HIV. HAART stands for "highly-active anti-retroviral therapy" and refers to combinations of three or more strong anti-HIV drugs that are taken together. These are often also referred to as "cocktail" drugs. HAART drugs are powerful and effective. In many people they can lower HIV in the blood so much that it can't be detected by blood tests. With the help of HAART, many people who were very sick with HIV improve and can often return to active, healthy lives. Others can take the medications to keep from ever getting sick in the first place.

That's the good part. The hard part is that these drug combinations do not work well for everyone. Sometimes there can be drug interactions, resistance, or side effects. And taking HAART can be difficult. Being on HAART means always taking at least three different HIV medications at the same time. Although some pills are now being made that combine two or more HAART drugs, so that taking them is easier, HAART is still a challenge. If you decide to be on HAART, it is very important that you take the medication regularly, as discussed with your doctor, without missing any doses.

People who do well taking HAART medications are those who understand that they won't always be easy to take, but who decide to take them anyway. All medications can have side effects in at least some of the people

---

[1] If you have access to the Internet it's a great idea to get familiar with a few reliable Web sites for HIV information. Several useful sites are listed at the end of this chapter.

who take them, and HAART medications are no exception. In Chapter 5, "Making Treatment Decisions," we discuss other issues to consider when making the decision to start on HAART therapy. In this chapter we describe the basics of HIV medications. We discuss side effects in Chapter 7, "Side Effects of Medications."

The number of anti-HIV HAART drugs available is growing every year. Once there were only a few different HAART medication combinations. Now there are many drugs, and hundreds of combinations. Guidelines for treating HIV all recommend that at least three anti-HIV drugs be used in combination whenever HAART is given.

The table at the end of this chapter lists the different HIV medications available when this book was published. There is more information out there about medications and treatment, much of it on the Internet. Our goal here is to give you a good starting point for talking with your doctor and doing more of your own research.

How HAART Medications Work

HIV lives in the body by making copies of itself, in a complicated series of chemical steps. If the virus *can't* copy itself, the immune system keeps it under control so that no HIV is detectable in the blood. As long as HIV isn't circulating in the blood, it can't damage the body. Anti-HIV HAART medications work by blocking the different steps the virus uses to copy itself. Here we discuss some of the different types of drugs that are part of HAART, what each of them does in the body, and the importance of taking them in combination.

Reverse transcriptase is one of the chemicals that occur naturally in the body, which HIV uses to copy itself. Many HIV drugs work by blocking reverse transcriptase. This is how *nucleoside* drugs such as zidovudine, lamivudine, and abacavir work. The drugs "fool" the reverse transcriptase into trying to use them as raw material to make HIV copies, and so they block the copying. Non-nucleoside reverse-transcriptase inhibitors (NNRTIs), such as nevirapine (Viramune) and efavirenz (Sustiva), work by binding to reverse transcriptase and blocking its action.

Protease is another of the body's naturally occurring chemicals that HIV uses fairly late in the process of copying itself. Drugs that block the protease

(*protease inhibitors*) are very powerful anti-HIV drugs and have become a crucial part of HAART combinations. Medications like nelfinavir (Viracept), indinavir (Crixivan), and saquinavir (Fortovase) are all protease inhibitors.

The newest class of HIV drugs is the *fusion inhibitor.* In order to copy itself and multiply in the body, HIV first has to *get inside* the human cell. Fusion inhibitors block the virus from ever getting into cells in the first place. The only approved HIV fusion inhibitor is enfuvirtide (Fuzeon), but others are being studied.

Drug Resistance and HIV

If all these drugs block the copying of HIV, why is it important to use two, three, or four different drugs at the same time? The reason is that HIV has the ability to become *resistant* to drugs. People who take only one single HIV drug can develop resistant HIV within months—or even weeks, in some cases. Once a person develops resistance to an HIV drug, that drug won't work against the person's resistant HIV. Because drug-resistant HIV can then be passed on to other people, it is a big problem not only for the person who has it, but also for people who may catch it from that person later.

HIV becomes resistant to a drug when the virus itself changes its structure so the drug can no longer attach, or otherwise can't do its work against the virus. How HIV does this is pretty complicated, but the good news is this: Even though HIV can become resistant to *one* drug, it can't become resistant to three, four, or more drugs *when they are taken at the same time.* It's almost as if the virus can only do its special "structure-changing" trick for one drug-enemy at a time. When facing many drugs, HIV just can't defend itself. This is why multi-drug HAART is so important, and why taking only one HIV drug and skipping your others is a bad idea.

Like the viral load and T cell tests discussed in Chapter 5, "Making Treatment Decisions" HIV drug resistance blood tests are important tools. Doctors use them to find out if a patient has drug-resistant HIV. Whether the person develops drug resistance, or catches a virus that is resistant from the start, the tests help doctors tell which HAART medications the HIV can respond to.

There are two main types of resistance tests. *Genotype tests* detect drug resistance mutations directly on the HIV genes. Genotype resistance tests give quick results, but they can be difficult to interpret and understand. In contrast, *phenotype tests* measure the HIV virus's ability to grow when exposed to different HAART drugs. It takes longer to get the results of phenotype tests, and they cost more than genotype tests, but they can still be helpful in some situations. In general, HIV resistance tests are most useful if a person has been taking HAART medications but the HIV is not responding. The tests may help tell you and your doctor *why* the HIV is not responding, and help with choosing a new, better HAART combination.

The Importance of Adherence

"Adherence" means that after you and your doctor have agreed on what medications to try, *you stick to taking the medications exactly as they are prescribed by the doctor*. If it is impossible to stick to the medications because of side effects or for some other reason, you need to talk about the problem with the doctor right away. It's very important to not miss any pills—whether by forgetting, intentionally skipping, lowering the dose, or changing the schedule.

There is so much information about HAART medications, and so many details to think about, that sometimes it's hard to see the big picture. These medicines have transformed HIV care, and they are very effective for many people. They may be effective for you—but they also require a big commitment. Taking HAART is work. Patients who choose to take HAART must take it consistently, without missing any doses. HAART can lead to side effects or drug resistance if not taken correctly. On the other hand, the benefits are real: People who take HAART correctly are much less likely to get AIDS-related infections and are much less likely to die. Many of them feel a lot stronger and healthier, too. HAART has revolutionized the lives of people with HIV.

Adhering to HIV medications can be difficult for all sorts of reasons. For one thing, HIV treatment plans are usually complicated. In research with people who have diseases that are much simpler than HIV (high blood pressure, for example), many people have difficulty adhering to even the simplest treatment plans. But HIV treatment is *not* simple. It sometimes involves taking twenty-five pills each day, or even more. And some HIV medications must be taken on an empty stomach, while others must be taken with meals. All this can be difficult, especially for people who are sick, weak, or experiencing severe HIV symptoms. To make it even more diffi-cult, HIV patients usually need to continue their treatments for the rest of their lives.

Side effects also can make it hard to stick with HIV treatment. Medications can cause problems like nausea, headaches, diarrhea, tiredness, or dizziness. Although it's much harder to stay on a medication that is caus-ing side effects, it's not impossible. Many side effects ease off with time or can be managed using simple techniques. Some of these techniques are dis-cussed in Chapter 7, "Side Effects of Medications."

For many people, the major problem with taking the medicines is that they just don't fit well into most daily routines. The medications aren't con-venient, so doses are forgotten. You may sleep through a dose, you may be away from home or be too busy, or you may simply forget.

Whether you're about to start HIV medications or you're already on HAART drugs, there are things you can do to make your treatment suc-cessful.

If you are considering starting HAART . . .

1. *Play an active role in the treatment plan.* Ask your doctor to describe all your options, including the potential benefits and risks of starting treat-ment now instead of later. Also ask your doctor to explain side effects or other problems that could be associated with the medication. If you're going to make the effort necessary to take these medications cor-rectly, you need to understand the goals of treatment and how to achieve them.

2. *Let your doctor know about personal issues that could make it hard for you to take the medications.* Be honest. Some things, such as use of drugs or alcohol, or problems with housing or mental illness, are not easy to talk about, but they should be discussed. Studies have shown that adherence to a treatment plan can be more difficult—but not impossible—for peo-ple dealing with drugs or alcohol or other personal problems. Adherence also may be more difficult for people who have very complex regimens or who have had problems taking medications in the past.

You can't always be sure what the problems are going to be. Many people do a "dry run," practicing the treatment using jelly beans or candy instead of real pills. This can help you anticipate what problems could arise.

3. *Ask for a written copy of the treatment plan.* It's helpful to have a list that shows each medication, when and how much to take each time, and whether it must be taken with food or on an empty stomach. Many doctors can give you a list that has pictures of the pills, so you won't get them confused.

4. Most important, *talk to your doctor about how to make your treatment fit your lifestyle.* For example, you might discuss how you can link the taking of medicines to certain things that you do each day—waking up in the morning, brushing your teeth, taking a child to school, leaving work, or watching a certain TV show. People who arrange their medication schedule around their daily routine adhere to their treatment plans better than those who don't.

5. *Make sure you can make a personal commitment to the treatment plan.* Talk to your doctor about all your concerns. You may need to talk things over two or three times before you feel comfortable about starting the anti-HIV drugs.

If you are already on HAART drugs and want to do better at taking them . . .

There are lots of strategies you can try, and it's vital that you find one that works for you. Here are some ideas:

1. *Try keeping your medications where you'll see them.* Some people find it helpful to keep their first morning dose next to the alarm clock or the coffee pot. Others keep backup medication supplies at work or in a briefcase.

2. *Use daily or weekly pillboxes to organize your medications.* Some people like to count and set out a week's medications at a time, with one box

or space for each part of the day. It often works well to count out pills at the same time each week, like every Sunday night at bedtime.

3. *Plan ahead for weekends, holidays, trips, and changes in routine.* Many studies have shown that weekends are a big problem for adherence. Decide ahead of time how you will remember to take all of your doses. Make a plan for remembering your medications, and write it out.

4. *Use timers, alarm clocks, pagers, or other tools to remind you when to take your medication.* There are a lot of tools out there, and one might work for you. For example, handheld computers like the Palm or BlackBerry, and some newer cell phones, can remind you to take your medicine. Take each medication at the same time every day.

5. *Keep a medication diary.* You can write the names of your drugs on a small card or in your daily planner, and then check off each dose as you take it.

6. *Get help and support from your family and friends.* You don't always have to go it alone. If you can, ask family members, friends, or loved ones to remind you to take your medication. Some people also find it helpful to join an HIV support group.

7. *Don't run out of medication.* Be sure to call your doctor or clinic if your supply won't last until your next visit.

HAART Medications for Pregnant Women with HIV

Women with HIV who are pregnant can pass the virus to their babies. But if they take antiretroviral medications while they are pregnant, the chance that the baby will get HIV is very low. It is very important for all women to get tested for HIV early in pregnancy, so that any woman who does have HIV can take medications to protect her baby.

Several different medication combinations can prevent passage of HIV from mother to child. Zidovudine + lamivudine has been used widely, as have nevirapine, and nevirapine + zidovudine. Other combinations may work well also. It is important to talk to your doctor and get good advice.

After the baby is born, the baby must also take anti-HIV medications for a while. By administering medication to both the pregnant mother and the new baby, HIV in newborn babies has been almost eliminated in the United States, Canada, and much of Europe. This is one of the biggest successes in HIV treatment worldwide.

PREVENTIVE MEDICATIONS

Even with good HAART medications available, specific antibiotics are still important for preventing opportunistic infections. (For more on opportunistic infections see Chapter 3, "Health Problems of People with HIV/AIDS.") Here we list some of the major AIDS opportunistic infections, along with descriptions of the medicines used to prevent and treat them.

Pneumocystis jiroveci (*Pneumocystis carinii*) Pneumonia (PCP)

Examples: Trimethoprim/sulfamethoxazole (Bactrim, Septra, TMP/SMX),[2] aerosolized pentamidine (NebuPent, AeroPent), dapsone, and dapsone + pyrimethamine + leukovorin. Atovaquone (Mepron) may also be an appropriate preventive medication for some people.

How they work: These medications all work by giving a steady, low dose of antibiotic to kill *Pneumocystis* before there are enough organisms to create a true pneumonia.

Possible side effects: With TMP/SMX, the most common side effect is an allergic skin reaction resulting in rashes, which can be successfully managed. Fair-skinned people on TMP/SMX are also sensitive to sunlight. Other side effects include minor fevers, nausea, low white blood cell count, decreased platelet count, and liver irritation. Dapsone is associated with less severe occurrence of nausea, vomiting, rashes, lowered red and white cell counts, and liver function problems. People with low levels of G6PD (a liver function

[2] Generic drug names are listed first, with alternative names for each drug in parentheses.

indicator) can develop rapid loss of blood cells on dapsone, so a G6PD test should be done before starting dapsone treatment. Aerosolized pentamidine is inhaled into the lungs rather than taken as a pill, so its most common side effect is a cough or raspy, dry throat, which can be minimized or eliminated by using inhaled medicines such as albuterol. Other side effects include a burning sensation in the back of the throat, an unpleasant taste, brief lung spasms, and (rarely) a mild decrease in blood sugar. Atovaquone has fewer side effects, but it is expensive.

Comments: TMP/SMX works extremely well for preventing PCP; almost no one who takes it regularly (daily or three times per week) comes down with the disease. The problem is that some people experience toxic reactions to TMP/SMX. These people may be able to take the medication if they take a gradually increasing dose, so that their bodies can get used to it. Otherwise, they should use one of the other medications.

Toxoplasmosis ("Toxo")

Examples: Trimethoprim/sulfamethoxazole (Bactrim, Septra, TMP/SMX), dapsone + pyrimethamine + leukovorin, clindamycin, and atovaquone (Mepron) are all used to prevent toxoplasmosis.

How they work: As with *Pneumocystis*, the idea is to kill the *Toxoplasma* organisms when they are present at microscopic levels, before they have started to actually invade the body. The medications all work by giving a steady low dose of antibiotic. Steady low doses are particularly important for people with a low CD4+ cell count and with a positive blood *Toxoplasma* antibody test.

Possible side effects: The side effects of TMP/SMX and dapsone are the same whether these drugs are used for toxoplasmosis or *Pneumocystis* prevention. Atovaquone has fewer side effects. Clindamycin causes rash and/or diarrhea in many people. Pyrimethamine can cause loss of red blood cells in some people but is well tolerated in most.

Comments: People who need toxoplasmosis prevention almost always need *Pneumocystis* prevention, too, so taking either TMP/SMX or dapsone can accomplish both goals. The other medications are less well proven but can be considered for a person who is taking aerosolized pentamidine to prevent *Pneumocystis* and therefore needs another medicine to prevent toxoplasmosis.

People need medications to prevent PCP and Toxo when their CD4+ cell count (T cell count) is lower than 200 per microliter. With HAART medications, many people can boost their immune systems so that their counts get above 200 and stay there. When this happens, they and their doctors may decide that they don't any longer need to take medicines to prevent PCP or Toxo. But of course they still need to stay on the HAART medications to keep the immune system strong, and they need to be tested regularly to make sure that the CD4+ cell count hasn't dropped back down below 200.

Tuberculosis (TB)

Examples: Isoniazid (INH) is the most common medicine for preventing TB disease in people who have a positive TB skin test. Rifampin or rifabutin and pyrazinamide may also be used. Still other drugs may be used if the doctor thinks you have been exposed to a drug-resistant form of TB. Depending on which medication or combination of medications is used, a person who has a positive TB skin test may need as little as 2 months or as much as 12 or more months of treatment to keep from getting TB disease.

How they work: If you're around someone with TB, a small number of organisms may get into your lungs and create a tiny infection. This is enough to make your immune system react and make your skin test positive, but it's not enough to cause disease. This is called latent TB infection. You've been *exposed* to TB, but you don't have *disease* from TB. The TB medications listed above, if taken correctly, can kill the TB organisms before they become active.

Possible side effects: INH can occasionally cause liver damage. It can also cause neuropathy (nerve damage in the arms and legs), but this problem is easy to prevent by taking vitamin B6 while you're on the INH.

Comments: The skin test for TB is very important because it can detect TB before it becomes active. Taking one medication to prevent TB disease is much better than waiting until the TB has spread to the lungs or other parts of the body. If TB becomes active in a person with HIV, usually at least four TB medications are needed to treat it. If the TB has gone too far, sometimes it can't be cured.

Mycobacterium avium Complex (MAC)

Examples: Azithromycin and Clarithromycin are effective for preventing MAC, and rifabutin is also sometimes used.

How they work: MAC is different from TB. There is no blood or skin test that can "catch" MAC when you've been exposed but are not yet actively infected. But we do know that the risk of MAC goes up sharply when the T cell count is below 100, and the risk is highest when the count is below 50. If a person has a low T cell count, taking azithromycin or clarithromycin can reduce the chances of getting MAC. These medicines work by killing the MAC before it gets a "foothold" in the body. As with PCP and Toxo, it may be possible to stop the MAC medication if HAART treatment makes the T cell count go above 100 and stay there.

Possible side effects: Clarithromycin and azithromycin can cause stomach upset or diarrhea, but generally they are well tolerated. Rifabutin may cause rashes, stomach upset, or a drop in the white blood cell count.

TREATMENT MEDICATIONS

Many of the medications described above for *preventing* problems seen in HIV/AIDS are also used for *treating* those problems when they occur. But treatment is always much more difficult. It requires higher doses, more medicines, and more complicated combinations, and it has more side effects. Many, many medications are used for treating different acute infections, so we will not discuss all of them here. Generally speaking, all exert their toxic effects to kill the invading virus, bacteria, parasite, or fungus, and all attempt to do this with minimal toxicity to the cells of the human body. Your treatment team should be your first source for information about medicines used to treat acute infections, but there are also other resources you can use. See the suggested resources list at the end of this chapter.

DECIDING WHEN TO TRY A NEW MEDICATION REGIMEN

Just like deciding when to start anti-HIV medications, deciding when to switch to a new combination of medicines is something that must be done very carefully, and always with the help of your doctor. Jumping from one set of medications to another too often can use up all your medication options, due to problems of resistance that we discussed earlier. But often, changing medications will be necessary, and this will be an important time for you to talk carefully with your doctor.

Although there are many factors to consider, in general there are two reasons why you might stop one set of anti-HIV medications and start another:

1. *Your current medications aren't working.* The job of the medications is to suppress the HIV in your blood, to boost or maintain your T cell count, and to keep you from getting HIV-related infections. If some of these things aren't being done well enough, it may be time to switch. This is pretty obvious, but what isn't so obvious is where to draw the line. How low should the viral load number be for your medicines to be considered successful? If your numbers have been low, how much of an increase should cause you to decide to make a change? How much of a drop in the T cell count should make you change? The main point to keep in mind is that if the numbers are going in the wrong direction (up

for viral load, down for T cells) and they're consistent on consecutive blood tests, then you and your doctor should talk about it. Depending on your situation, either staying on your medication or switching to a new combination may be the right decision.

2. *Your current medications are too toxic.* It could be that your anti-HIV drugs are suppressing HIV very well and boosting your T cells, but that one or more of the drugs is making you so sick that you have to change. If you find this happening to you, talk with your doctor right away. Otherwise, you may wind up skipping or "forgetting" doses, and put yourself at risk for resistance. Only you know what your side effects are like and whether they're severe enough to warrant a change of medications. Although there are more treatment options now than ever before, the choices are still limited in many cases, so it's important to balance side effects against benefits when you make your decision.

In the next chapter we discuss some common side effects of the medications we introduced here.

EVALUATING TREATMENTS

Besides the treatments listed in this book, you will no doubt hear of many other treatments. Some of them may be exciting new medicines developed after this book was printed. Others will be attempts to sell you useless products. In evaluating any treatment—whether it's a new medication, a non-traditional "alternative" treatment, or even a surgical procedure—there are some key questions to ask yourself and others.

- **Is there proof?** Does the report about the effectiveness of the treatment come from a scientific study, or from a story you heard from an individual or from the marketer of the treatment?

- **If the proof was from a scientific study, was there a control group?** In a scientific research project, there should be a group of people, called the control group, who don't receive the treatment and are compared to the group that does receive the treatment. For example, one group may get a new medication while the control group gets a sugar pill. This same method is used to study the effectiveness of any treatment. Without a control group, there is no reliable way to determine whether good results are due to the treatment or to something else.

- **Were the people who benefited from the treatment like me?** Were they the same gender, lifestyle, and age, and in the same state of health? If not, the results may not apply to your situation.

- **Could anything else have caused the results?** Was there a seasonal change, other medication, emotional changes, a change in lifestyle, or any other factor that could have caused the people in the study to feel better?

- **Where were the results published?** Did they appear in a reputable scientific journal or Web site, or in a supermarket tabloid?

- **Does this treatment require me to eliminate other treatments or foods?** The new treatment may have serious interactions with the treatments you are already taking. Does the new plan stress only a few nutrients or foods, and perhaps leave you without other nutrients that you need?

- **Are there any possible dangers?** Ask your doctor, pharmacist, or other health professionals about the treatment. Remember, too, that "natural" doesn't mean that something is safe. Dosages of "natural" products may not be well controlled, and are usually not regulated.

- **Can I afford it?** Can you afford it—financially, physically, and emotionally?

- **Am I willing to take the trouble?** New treatments often take effort, time, and resources. Do you have the necessary support to maintain the new treatment?

Once you have answered these questions and have decided to try a new treatment, make sure to keep your doctor and other members of your health care team informed.

HIGHLY ACTIVE ANTIRETROVIRAL THERAPY (HAART) DRUGS[3]

Generic Name (Abbreviation)	Formulations	Usual Adult Doses	Food Effects	Common Side Effects
Nucleoside Reverse Transcriptase Inhibitors (NRTIs)				
Abacavir (ABC)	Ziagen Trizivir (with ZDV +3TC) Epzicom (with 3TC)	300 mg 2 tims/day; or 600 mg once daily	Take without regard to meals Alcohol increases abacavir levels	Nausea, vomiting, headache, fatigue. A small number of people develop hypersensitivity, with flu-like symptoms. If this happens, stop the drug immediately and tell the doctor.
Didanosine (ddI)	Videx Videx EC	Body weight ≥60 kg: 400 mg once daily (buffered tablets or EC capsule); or 200 mg two times/day (buffered tablets); Body weight <60 kg: 250 mg daily (buffered tablets or EC capsule); or 125 mg two times/day (buffered tablets)	Take ½ hour before or 2 hours after meal	Increased uric acid levels, headaches, sleepiness, diarrhea, pain or tingling in the feet or hands.

[3] Adapted from *Guidelines for the Use of Antiretroviral Agents in HIV-1-Infected Adults and Adolescents*, developed by the panel on Clinical Practices for Treatment of HIV Infection convened by the Department of Health and Human Services (DHHS) and the Henry J. Kaiser Family Foundation, October 29, 2004.

Nucleoside Reverse Transcriptase Inhihibitors (NRTIs)

Generic Name (Abbreviation)	Formulations	Usual Adult Doses	Food Effects	Common Side Effects
Emtricitabine (FTC)	Emtriva Truvada (with TDF)	200 mg once daily	Take without regard to meals	Rash, diarrhea, headache, nausea, vomiting
Lamivudine (3TC)	Epivir Combivir (with ZDV) Epizicom (with ABC) Trizivir (with ZDV +ABC)	150 mg two times/day; or 300 mg daily	Take without regard to meals	Headaches, nausea, sense of feeling ill, diarrhea, anemia, hair loss
Stavudine (d4T)	Zerit	Body weight >60 kg: 40 mg two times/day; Body weight <60 kg: 30 mg two times/day	Take without regard to meals	Pain or tingling in the feet or hands, anemia. Rarely, pancreatitis can occur. Symptoms include pain in the abdomen, nausea vomiting. The drug must be stopped immediately and doctor contacted.

Generic Name (Abbreviation)	Formulations	Usual Adult Doses	Food Effects	Common Side Effects
Nucleoside Reverse Transcriptase Inhihibitors (NRTIs)				
Tenofovir Disoproxil Fumarate (TDF)	Viread Truvada (with FTC)	300 mg tablet once daily	Take without regard to meals	Nausea, diarrhea, vomiting, flatulence, rash
Zalcitabine (ddC)	Hivid	0.75 mg three times/day	Take without regard to meals	Pain or tingling in the feet or hands, oral ulcers, low platelets. Rarely, pancreatitis (see stavudine above).
Zidovudine (AZT, ZDV)	Retrovir Combivir (with 3TC) Trizivir (with 3TC + ABC)	300 mg two times/day or 200 mg three times/day	Take without regard to meals	Headache, nausea, sense of feeling ill, anemia

Non-Nucleoside Reverse Transcriptase Inhihibitors (NNRTIs)

Generic Name (Abbreviation)	Formulations	Usual Adult Doses	Food Effects	Common Side Effects
Delavirdine (DLV)	Rescriptor	400 mg 3 times/day; avoid taking within an hour of taking buffered didanosine or antacids	Take without regard to meals	Rash, which usually appears within the first 3 weeks of treatment.
Efavirenz (EFV)	Sustiva	600 mg daily on an empty stomach, at or before bedtime	High-fat/high-calorie food can make drug levels too high in the blood; take on an empty stomach	Neurological symptoms such as dizziness, drowsiness, and lack of concentration.
Nevirapine (NVP)	Viramune	200 mg daily for 14 days; thereafter, 200 mg by mouth two times/day	Take without regard to meals	Rash, which usually appears within the first 3 weeks of treatment.

Protease Inhibitors (PIs)

Generic Name (Abbreviation)	Formulations	Usual Adult Doses	Food Effects	Common Side Effects
Atazanavir (ATV)	Reyataz	400 mg once daily; or (300 mg ATV + 100 mg RTV) once daily	Take with food; avoid taking with antacids	Nausea, headache, rash, vomiting, diarrhea.
Fosamprenavir (f-APV)	Lexiva	1400 mg two times/day; or (700 mg f-APV + 100 mg RTV) two times/day; or (1400 mgs f-APV + 200 mg RTV) once daily	Take without regard to meals.	Diarrhea, headache, nausea, vomiting, depression, abdominal pain, rash

Generic Name (Abbreviation)	Formulations	Usual Adult Doses	Food Effects	Common Side Effects
Protease Inhihibitors (PIs)				
Indinavir (IDV)	Crixivan	800 mg every 8 hours or may boost concentrations in blood by dosing with RTV —discuss with doctor.	For RTV-boosted IDV: Take with or without food. For unboosted IDV: Take 1 hour before or 2 hours after meals; may take with skim milk or low-fat meal.	Kidney stones. Drink at least 8 glasses of water per day to reduce this risk.
Lopinavir + Ritonavir (LPV/r)	Kaletra	[LPV 400 mg + RTV 100 mg] (3 capsules or 5 milliliters) two times daily	Moderate-fat meal increases concentration. Take with food.	Diarrhea, nausea, high blood lipids, headache

Protease Inhihibitors (PIs)

Generic Name (Abbreviation)	Formulations	Usual Adult Doses	Food Effects	Common Side Effects
Nelfinavir	Viracept	1250 mg two times/day or 750 mg three times/day	Take with meal or snack	Diarrhea and nausea
Ritonavir (RTV)	Norvir	600 mg every 12 hours (when ritonavir is used as sole PI). When used to boost the blood levels of other PIs: 100 mg– 400 mg per day, in 1–2 divided doses	Take with food if possible; this may reduce side effects	Diarrhea and nausea, which are usually worse in the first few weeks of starting the medication

Generic Name (Abbreviation)	Formulations	Usual Adult Doses	Food Effects	Common Side Effects
		Protease Inhihibitors (PIs)		
Saquinavir hard gel capsule (SQV-hgc)	Invirase	Unboosted SQV-hgc is not recommended With RTV: (RTV 100 mg + SQV-hgc 1000 mg) two times/day (RTV 400 mg + SQV-hgc 400 mg) two times/day	Take within 2 hours of a meal with RTV	Diarrhea and nausea
Saquinavir soft capsule (SQV-sgc)	Fortovase	Unboosted SQV-sgc: 1200 mg three times/day	Take with a meal or up to 2 hours after eating	Diarrhea and nausea

Generic Name (Abbreviation)	Formulations	Usual Adult Doses	Food Effects	Common Side Effects
Protease Inhihibitors (PIs)				
Saquinavir (cont.)	Fortovase	With RTV: (RTV 100 mg + SQV-sgc 1000 mg) two times/day RTV 400 mg + SQV-sgc 400 mg two times/day		
Fusion Inhihibitors				
Enfuvirtide (T20)	Fuzeon	Inject 90 mg (1 mL) subcutaneously (SC) two times/day	N/A	Injection site reactions, diarrhea, nausea, fatigue, insomnia

SUGGESTED RESOURCES FOR MORE INFORMATION ABOUT MEDICATIONS

Books

Bartlett, John G., and Finkbeiner, Ann K. *The Guide to Living with HIV Infection*, developed at The Johns Hopkins AIDS Clinic. 5th ed. Baltimore, Md.: The Johns Hopkins University Press, 2001.

Grodeck, Brett. *The First Years—HIV: An Essential Guide for the Newly Diagnosed*. Foreword by Daniel S. Berger. New York: Marlowe, 2003.

Rybacki, James J., and Long, James W. *The Essential Guide to Prescription Drugs*. New York: Harper Resource, 2004.

Silverman, Harold. *The Pill Book*. 11th ed. New York: Bantam Doubleday, 2004.

The Internet

The Internet is one of the best places to get up-to-date information about HIV. The following sites are good places to start:

The Body: AIDS and HIV Information Resource
www.thebody.com/index.shtml

HIVInSite
hivinsite.ucsf.edu/medical

AIDS Info: U.S. Dept. of Health and Human Services
aidsinfo.nih.gov/ed_resources

AMFAR Global Link HIV treatment information
web.amfar.org/treatment/index.asp

Project Inform: nonprofit, HIV community-based organization
projinf.org/

Telephone Information

Centers for Disease Control (CDC) HIV/AIDS Treatment Information Service
(800) 448-0440

National Institutes of Health (NIH) AIDS Clinical Trials Information Service
(800) TRIALS-A

Project Inform Treatment Hotline
(800) 822-7422

CHAPTER SEVEN

Side Effects of Medications

Medication side effects are a very big issue in HIV treatments. Nowadays, managing the side effects of HAART can be almost as big a part of care as managing HIV itself. But there are many good ways to manage side effects, and managing them is crucial because HAART medications are so crucial. This chapter will provide you with information that will help you to identify, cope with, and self-manage these side effects.

Most side effects are predictable and minor, but some can be serious. Sometimes hospital admissions are necessary because of side effects. In spite of this, there's no reason to be frightened of medications. By knowing what medications you're using, knowing what (and what not) to expect, and getting proper checkups and tests, you can maximize your benefit and reduce the chances of serious side effects.

WHAT IS A SIDE EFFECT?

A side effect is any effect a medication has other than the one you want. Usually, it is an undesirable effect. Examples of undesirable side effects are stomach problems, constipation, diarrhea, sleepiness, and dizziness. You should know the common side effects of the medications you take.

Patients and doctors have to figure out how to manage side effects and how to decide when they are dangerous, when they will improve on their own, and when they are so bothersome that the medications should be changed. Luckily, many side effects can be managed, so you won't have to stop using a medication and give up its benefits.

QUESTIONS TO ASK ABOUT SIDE EFFECTS

Sometimes people say they can't or won't take a drug because of its possible side effects. This is understandable. However, before you make a decision to stop taking a drug or refuse to take it, you should ask yourself and your doctor the following questions.

Are the benefits from this medication more important than the side effects?
HAART drugs are a good example of medications whose benefits should be weighed against their undesirable side effects. Although these drugs have side effects, many people still take them because of their life-saving qualities. To start or not start the drugs is your decision. However, you should always ask yourself, "*Even with* the side effects, will I be better off with the drugs than I would be without them?" With HAART, it's also important to remember that a decision you make today may be different from the decision you make later on. For example, if you're healthy now, you and your doctor may decide that starting HAART now isn't worth it. But later on, you might make a very different decision if you're not feeling as well and your T cells are lower. See Chapter 5, "Making Treatment Decisions," for more guidance on making decisions about this important treatment option.

Is the problem I'm having *really* a medication side effect?
Sometimes it is easy to tell whether a symptom you're having is a side effect from a medication, but other times it can be hard. You might think, for example, that a new headache, stomachache, or other symptom is being caused by your medication. But the symptom may be temporary, or be caused by something different. Before you make a permanent change, it's important to discuss these issues with your provider.

Are there ways of avoiding the side effects or making them less severe?

Many times, the *way* you take the drug—for example, with or without food—can make a difference. Several self-management strategies for side effects are included in this book. Ask your doctor or pharmacist for advice, too.

Are there other medications that have the same benefits, but fewer side effects?

Several different drugs may be designed to treat the same medical problem, and they may have different side effects in different people. Unfortunately, you cannot know how you will react to a drug until you have taken it. Therefore, your doctor may have to try several different medications before hitting on the ones that are best for you.

COMMON SIDE EFFECTS OF HIV/AIDS MEDICATIONS

The effects and side effects of HIV medications can be complicated. It may be tough to figure out how to minimize the side effects and still get the benefits you need. Your doctor, nurse, and pharmacist are your main resources for advice about your medications, and you need to talk to them whenever you think of making a change. There are lots of other places to get helpful information, too. Some information about lipodystrophy, high blood sugar, and high cholesterol is included here. See the accompanying table, "Techniques for Managing Side Effects," for more on other common side effects.

You will also find information about medication-specific side effects in the table at the end of Chapter 6, "Managing Medications for HIV/AIDS." That table lists some of the other side effects that have been associated with anti-HIV medications and gives some self-management techniques to try. Even if you have success in managing your side effects, remember to keep your doctors and nurses informed about new side effects—especially any severe ones. You should also check the symptom action charts in Chapter 8, "Evaluating Common Symptoms of HIV/AIDS," which can help you determine whether a symptom is a side effect or a sign of a serious illness.

Fat Redistribution (Lipodystrophy)

People getting treatment for HIV can have changes in the way fat is distributed on their bodies. Their bodies may gradually start to look different. Doctors call this *lipodystrophy*. The changes are difficult to describe exactly, but usually *more* fat goes to the central part of the body (the stomach, the breasts, the upper back), and *less* fat remains in the face, rear end, and arms and legs. Women's breasts may get very large due to fatty deposits, which causes real problems with comfort and clothing. People with lipodystrophy may start to see prominent veins on their legs or they may notice changes in their faces as a result of the fat loss. These changes can be accompanied by changes in cholesterol and blood sugar levels so they should not be ignored. In some cases, lipodystrophy can make people feel ugly or self-conscious, and may reduce their quality of life. In other cases it is pretty mild, and feels like a good trade-off for the big benefits of HIV treatment.

Doctors are not certain exactly what causes lipodystrophy. It may be a side effect from taking protease inhibitors. However, it sometimes occurs in people not taking these drugs and even in people who have never used an anti-HIV drug. Although anyone with HIV can have lipodystrophy, it is probably more common in people using protease inhibitor medications.

Whatever the cause, the changes in appearance can be upsetting for some people, and some may even decide to stop taking their HIV medications because of the changes. But people who discontinue HAART medications for any reason must discuss it with their doctors. They will need a different program of laboratory tests, and may also need to take other medications in order to avoid HIV-related infections.

Exercise and gradual, healthy weight loss may help reduce lipodystrophy in some people. Exercise to build muscle has been found effective in studies. Please see Chapter 11, "Exercising for Fun and Fitness," for more about how exercise can help this condition. Some people have cosmetic surgery to remove fat or to fill in places where fat has been lost, but this is a costly approach and is not available to everyone. There are also new medications being tested to treat lipodystrophy, but we will need to wait and see what research on these will show.

High Cholesterol and High Blood Sugar

High levels of cholesterol and sugar in the blood are conditions that may be caused by a person's diet, or they may run in some families. They're a problem for lots of people, and that's why you see ads on TV and in magazines for cholesterol and blood sugar treatments. People with HIV can also have higher cholesterol and blood sugar levels. In addition, HAART also increases the risk of high blood sugar and cholesterol. Because of this, people taking HAART may have a higher risk of heart disease. For most people with HIV, it still makes sense to use HAART to control HIV. While they are on HAART medications, however, people need to take steps to lower blood sugar and cholesterol to reduce the risk of heart disease. If a person on HAART has large enough increases in blood sugar, they may develop diabetes. If diabetes develops, it may be necessary to use prescription medications to reduce cholesterol or lower the blood sugar. Chapter 12, "Healthy Eating," provides some tips on how to cut back on fat and sugar in the diet. People with high blood cholesterol or blood sugar may want to use these tips to change their eating habits.

If you're a smoker (and especially a smoker who takes HAART drugs), the best way to lower your heart disease risk is to stop smoking. You will also want to keep your blood pressure at a healthy level, eat a healthy diet, and exercise. All these things will lower your chances of heart disease, and you'll find tips about them in the chapters in Part 4, "Managing Exercise and Diet."

TECHNIQUES FOR MANAGING SIDE EFFECTS	
Diarrhea	This is a very common side effect, especially in the first few weeks of taking a new medication. It often goes away on its own. • Eat frequent, small meals. • Eat plenty of fiber (vegetables) and drink lots of liquids (water, juice, caffeine-free beverages). • Eat rice and other starches, oatmeal, potatoes, apples (peeled and allowed to brown), pears, bananas. • Avoid dairy products (milk, ice cream, cheese), caffeine, fast foods, fried foods. • Consider switching to a low-fat diet. • Consider adding acidophilus (from a health food or drug store) to your diet. Share your plan to take acidophilus with your doctor or nurse beforehand, to make sure it does not interfere with the rest of your treatment plan. • When going away from home, make sure bathrooms will be available. • Consider taking extra underpants with you if you will be away from home for a long time. • Ask your doctor about Metamucil, Lomotil, Imodium, or tincture of opium. • **Keep your doctor or primary care provider informed**.
Fatigue	This is a very common side effect, especially in the first few weeks of taking a new medication. It often goes away on its own. • Take frequent, short naps and try to sleep longer at night. • Limit caffeine and sugar. • Limit work hours, if possible. • Try relaxation techniques.[*]

[*] Relaxation techniques are described in Chapter 10, "Using Your Mind to Manage Symptoms." Many bookstores have books or audio tapes or CDs that can assist you.

TECHNIQUES FOR MANAGING SIDE EFFECTS (CONTINUED)

Fatigue
- Participate in light exercise (e.g., 15 to 30 minutes of brisk walking).
- **Keep your doctor or primary care provider informed.**

"Feeling different"
Many patients feel different, as if their thinking process or perception of the world has changed. Some will feel almost as if they're dreaming. This is a very common side effect, especially in the first few weeks of a regimen. It often goes away on its own.
- Try relaxation techniques.*
- Increase your sleep time and try short naps.
- Avoid alcohol and other drugs.
- Participate in light exercise (e.g., 15 to 30 minutes of brisk walking).
- **Keep your doctor or primary care provider informed.**

Dizziness
This is a common side effect, but can also be a symptom due to a new medical problem. Therefore, **your first step is to have new dizziness evaluated by your doctor or nurse.** If it's not a sign of a serious problem, it may go away on its own.
- Sit down and put your head between your knees, or lie down with your feet higher than your head.
- Drink plenty of liquids (water, juice, caffeine-free beverages).
- Rise slowly when waking up—sit up first.
- Eat high-energy foods.
- When indoors, make sure you have enough fresh air.
- Loosen tight-fitting clothing.
- Avoid alcohol and other drugs.
- **Keep your doctor or primary care provider informed.**

TECHNIQUES FOR MANAGING SIDE EFFECTS (CONTINUED)

Headache   This is a very common side effect, especially in the first few weeks of taking a new medication. It often goes away on its own.

- Take Tylenol, aspirin, or Advil.
- Try relaxation techniques,* herbal teas, soft music.
- **Keep your doctor or primary care provider informed.**

Nausea   This is a very common side effect, especially in the first few weeks of taking a new medication. It often goes away on its own.

- Eat crackers, and sip ginger ale or other soft drinks.
- Eat cold or room-temperature foods and liquids.
- Avoid odors, sights, or sounds that trigger the nausea.
- Avoid greasy foods, fried foods, alcohol.
- Breathe in fresh air, or pleasant smells such as lemon or lime peels and ginger.
- Try Mylanta or Maalox (but not at the same time you take your HIV medications).
- Avoid spicy foods and foods with lots of acid (e.g., oranges, tomatoes).
- Ask your doctor about Zofran, Compazine, and benzodiazepines.
- **Keep your doctor or primary care provider informed.**

If you are using didanosine (ddI):
- Try crushing and dissolving pills in ice-cold water or juice.
- Try taking pills at a different time (like at bedtime).
- Remember that ddI must be taken on an empty stomach.

---

*Relaxation techniques are described in Chapter 10, "Using Your Mind to Manage Symptoms." Many bookstores have books or audio tapes or CDs that can assist you.

TECHNIQUES FOR MANAGING SIDE EFFECTS (CONTINUED)

Numbness or tingling
This is a very common side effect, which can go away on its own.
- Eat a balanced diet and take a multivitamin each day.
- Tell your doctor or primary care provider if there is an increase in numbness or in the size of the numb area.
- Do passive flexibility exercises with your hands/arms/legs/feet; ask a family member or friend to assist.
- Massage your hands/arms/legs/feet.
- Wear loose-fitting, comfortable shoes with padded soles.

Rash
This is a very common side effect, especially in the first few weeks of taking a new medication. It can go away on its own, **but it is very important that you see your doctor.**
- Talk to your doctor or primary care provider to get "urgent" care for new rashes.
- Air- or pat-dry your skin after bathing.
- Apply moisturizing creams or lotions that do not contain alcohol.
- Wear light, non-irritating clothing and a hat when in the sun.
- Keep sheets and blankets off sensitive skin (e.g., use a pillow at the foot of the bed to hold sheets off your feet).
- Try not to scratch. Keep your fingernails short and clean.
- Report increasing rash, fever, headache, flu-like symptoms, or any sores in your mouth or vagina.
- Benadryl may help with itching (but **use it only** with your doctor's approval).

PART THREE

Managing Symptoms and Long-Term Health

CHAPTER EIGHT

Evaluating Common Symptoms of HIV/AIDS

Symptoms are the body's signals that something unusual is happening, that something is not right. They cannot always be seen by others, are often difficult to describe, and are usually unpredictable. If you have HIV/AIDS you are probably going to have symptoms that will need to be managed. Although some symptoms are common, when and how they affect each of us is very personal. Also, symptoms such as fatigue, stress, shortness of breath, pain, anger, depression, and sleep disturbances can interact with each other, which in turn worsens health and leads to the development of new symptoms.

Although the chronic symptoms that people with HIV/AIDS get are difficult to live with, there are many things you can do to deal successfully with them. In this chapter we look at how to evaluate some of the common symptoms associated with HIV/AIDS so that you can decide whether a symptom needs immediate medical attention. If you have not experienced any symptoms, this information will help prepare you for what to expect if symptoms do begin. It will also help you determine whether symptoms are part of a normal illness, such as a common cold or the flu, or something more serious. In Chapter 9 we discuss the more common chronic symptoms of HIV/AIDS and some of their causes, and in Chapter 10 we present some specific suggestions and techniques that involve the use of the mind for dealing with these symptoms.

SYMPTOM TYPES

In general, people with HIV/AIDS can view their symptoms as falling into three broad groups.

First, some symptoms are medication side effects—symptoms caused by the medications themselves. We discuss side effects and some management strategies in Chapter 7, "Side Effects of Medications," and you will also find additional medication-specific information in the table at the end of Chapter 6, "Managing Medications for HIV/AIDS."

Second, new symptoms could be caused by a new HIV-related infection. For example, a new cough with fever could be a symptom of pneumonia. People who have symptoms that might be from new infections need to see the doctor right away, because detecting these conditions and starting treatment early is vital. The symptom action charts included later in this chapter are designed to help people decide when it's important to see the doctor.

Third, many chronic conditions (including chronic HIV) can cause symptoms themselves. People with arthritis may get joint or back pains, people with chronic lung disease may become short of breath, and people with HIV may develop fatigue or other symptoms. Chronic symptoms may increase and decrease but they can be managed with a good program for living well.

SYMPTOM MANAGEMENT BASICS

In addition to helping you deal with your disease symptoms, the various techniques described throughout this book will also help you live well by maintaining health and slowing or preventing the onset of new symptoms.

Keep the following suggestions in mind when trying out a self-management technique and planning your self-management program:

- *Read all three chapters on symptoms and their management* (Chapters 8–10).

- *Evaluate each new symptom.* Symptoms are always distressing but sometimes they are also important clues that something new is happening that needs to be addressed. A new or worsening symptom could be a sign of a drug side effect or an opportunistic infection. (See Chapter 3, "Health Problems of People with HIV/AIDS," for more on opportunistic infections.) To be an effective self-manager, you need to know when it's okay to use home self-management techniques and when you should see the doctor.

- *Pick one technique to try first.* Be sure to give it a fair trial. We recommend that you practice the technique for at least two weeks, twice a day, before deciding whether it is going to be helpful. Also try some of the other techniques, giving each the same trial period. It is important to try more than one technique, because some may be more useful for a particular symptom, or you may find that you simply prefer some techniques over others.

- *After choosing the techniques you like, think about how and when you will use each one.* This will depend on exactly what you're trying to accomplish. Some techniques are specific to certain symptoms. For example, certain diet changes may be appropriate for managing diarrhea, whereas inhaling moist heat is good for nasal congestion. Some of the exercises can be done anywhere; others require a quiet place. Some may require substantial lifestyle changes. You may find in your practice of the different techniques that some work well for certain symptoms but not so well for others. The best symptom managers learn to use a variety of techniques tailored to their needs and situations.

- *Finally, because practice and consistency are important for the mastery of some of these techniques, place cues in your environment to remind you to practice them.* For example, place a sticker or note where you'll see it, such as on your mirror, in your office, next to your medicines, on the car's dashboard, or near your home phone. You can change the stickers or notes periodically so you will continue to notice them. Also, try linking these new activities to some other established behavior or activity in your daily routine. For example, practice relaxation as part of your cooldown after exercise. You might ask a friend, family member, or partner to remind you to get your practice in each day; they may even wish to participate.

EVALUATING YOUR SYMPTOMS

One of the most difficult things about living with HIV is that one is always concerned about developing an AIDS-related infection or other condition. New symptoms, especially if they are your first symptoms, are distressing in and of themselves. They are also distressing because they could be signals of a new or more serious problem. The truth is that symptoms can sometimes be signals that a serious illness is starting, for which you should see your doctor. Just as often, however, the symptoms are part of the cycle of chronic disease, for which self-management may be the best approach (see Figure 1.1 on page 6).

To feel confident in using self-management, you need to know when it's time to call the doctor. But how can you tell? Some of it is common sense. If it's clear you're having a medical emergency, see a doctor immediately. On the other hand, if you're having symptoms similar to what you've often had in the past, you can probably use self-management techniques confidently.

Another important factor in evaluating symptoms is to know your T cell count (also called CD4+ cell count). T cells are one way of estimating the strength of the immune system; people with a T cell count lower than 200 are usually at higher risk for getting infections, so they have to be more careful. Your doctor should measure your T cell count at least every six months, and often every three months. It's a good idea to know the result of your most recent measurement. Of course, T cells aren't the only measure of how healthy you are, although they are useful. There's more information about T cell counts in Chapter 5, "Making Treatment Decisions."

One quick way to judge whether you should see your doctor for a symptom is to do a "FAST" check. The initials in the acronym "FAST" stand for Fever, Altered mental status, Severe, and Typical. Ask yourself the four simple questions listed in the following chart. If the answer to any of the questions is yes, you should see your doctor promptly. He or she will be able to tell you if the symptom is due to a new AIDS-related infection or cancer.

Fever

Fever can be a chronic symptom in advanced HIV/AIDS, but it also can be an important clue when it appears in association with another symptom. A temperature of 101°F (38.3°C) is more likely to be associated with infection. Everyone with HIV needs to own, and know how to use, a thermometer. It is important to measure your temperature when you think you have a fever. Write down the temperature so you will be able to tell the doctor if necessary.

DO A FAST CHECK ON ALL NEW OR WORSENING SYMPTOMS

Fever   Is the new symptom associated with a fever (a temperature of 101°F or more)?

Altered mental status   Is the new symptom associated with an alteration in your mental status (e.g., confusion, sleepiness, seizures)?

Severe   Is the new symptom much more severe than anything you've had in the past?

Typical   Is the new symptom not typical for you?

Altered Mental Status

The brain is the body's most important organ, so it is a sensitive indicator of when trouble is present. *Altered mental status* is a term doctors use to describe a person whose brain functioning is not normal. This can mean confusion, excessive sleepiness, or "I can't put my finger on it, but he just isn't himself." It can also take a much more dramatic form, such as a coma (the most extreme decrease in mental function) or a seizure. All of these conditions represent altered mental states. Anyone who develops altered mental status over a short period of time, particularly in association with other symptoms, should see a doctor promptly.

You may not be able to recognize a serious alteration in mental function yourself, but you can teach those close to you how to easily diagnose such a change. If they suspect you may be subject to an altered mental status, they should simply see how well you answer questions. If you can't answer questions coherently or can't wake up enough to answer them, urgent action is needed.

Severe

Chronic symptoms will often increase and decrease depending on whether you're having a good day or a bad day. However, any symptom that is much more severe than it has ever been before should be evaluated by your health care team.

Typical

Any symptom that is completely new for you (that is, *not* typical) should be discussed with your medical team. This is a very general guideline that you probably use already when deciding whether to go to the doctor. Depending on what the new symptom is, you may want to consult one of the symptom action charts that follow for more guidance. But remember that when in doubt, it's better to be safe than sorry. If you're experiencing a symptom you've never had before and you're not sure whether self-care is the right thing to do, it's best to consult your doctor to be sure.

USING SYMPTOM ACTION CHARTS

Another way to evaluate your symptoms is to use action charts. These charts will guide you in evaluating several common HIV/AIDS-related symptoms that sometimes require a doctor's rapid attention. Not every symptom is included here, but if you have one of the symptoms listed, the chart will help you decide what to do.

If you have more than one symptom, you may need to look at more than one chart. If the advice in the two charts doesn't agree, follow the most "conservative" (that is, the safest) advice. For example, if one chart says to call the doctor and the other recommends home treatment, you should call your doctor.

If you use the charts properly by following the steps below, they will guide you through the key questions you should consider in deciding whether you need the help of your health care team right away.

1. *Determine your "chief complaint" or symptom*, and then find the correct chart. (They are arranged alphabetically.)

2. Before you look at the chart, *read the general text information on the symptom, which accompanies the chart*. This information will help you understand the questions in the chart. If you ignore the general information, you may not understand the questions in the chart correctly, and you could do the wrong thing.

3. *Read the action chart.* Start at the top and follow the arrows. Skipping around may result in errors. Each question assumes that you have answered all of the previous questions.

   Note: These charts are intended only to help you decide whether you urgently need to see your doctor for certain symptoms. Regardless of symptoms, you should always get the routine checkups that you and your doctor have scheduled.

COUGH

The cough reflex is a defense mechanism used by the body to clear abnormal material from the lungs. When the cough is bringing up infected material, such as pus, from the lungs, coughing is beneficial and shouldn't be suppressed. However, anything that irritates the lungs will cause a cough, and many of these stimuli do not produce pus, or even anything that's particularly easy to get out. So the cough will continue but not produce anything, which can be quite aggravating.

A cough can be a medication side effect, but the medications most commonly associated with this are for blood pressure or heart disease (captopril, fosinopril, lisinopril, enalapril, benazopril). For most people with HIV, a new cough is related to something else.

People with HIV/AIDS get coughs for all the same reasons other people do. Smoking is probably the most common cause; the toxins in the smoke irritate and kill cells in the lining of the bronchial tubes (breathing tubes) and stimulate the cough. This can happen even to those who don't

---

COUGH ACTION CHART

Is the cough associated with *shortness of breath at rest* or upon *minimal exertion?*   **Yes** → See doctor now.

No ↓

Is the *cough dry* and associated with *fever?*   **Yes** → See doctor today.

No ↓

Is the cough associated with *fever* and *pain in the chest?*   **Yes** → See doctor today.

No ↓

Is the cough producing thick, foul-smelling, *rusty or greenish mucus?*   **Yes** → See doctor today.

No ↓

Has *fever* lasted more than 4 days or has cough lasted more than 10 days?   **Yes** → Make appointment with doctor.

No ↓

Home treatment (see page 117)

themselves smoke but who breathe other people's smoke. Viral infections ("colds") are the next most common cause. These coughs usually produce only yellow or whitish mucus, not the green or rusty stuff produced by a more serious bacterial infection. Cold viruses don't respond to antibiotics; the only treatment for them is to strengthen the body's immune response with rest, good food, and lots of fluids. Bacterial infections can be more serious and require a doctor's attention and antibiotics.

In addition to the usual causes of cough, people with HIV/AIDS are susceptible to lung diseases not usually seen in people with stronger immune systems. The most common and most important of these is *Pneumocystis* pneumonia (PCP). Identifying this disease early is vital because it is very dangerous when advanced. When caught early, however, it responds very well to antibiotics. The signs of PCP are a dry cough with shortness of breath and fever. Other lung infections that are seen in people with HIV/AIDS include tuberculosis (TB) and bacterial pneumonia. TB is a very serious lung disease that may cause a chronic cough with fevers, yet may not cause much trouble with breathing. Unfortunately, TB is very easy to pass on to other people by coughing. Because of the risk of TB, you should bring any persistent cough (lasting longer than ten days) to the attention of your doctor. See Chapter 3, "Health Problems of People with HIV/AIDS," for more on these illnesses.

Infection in the sinuses (sinusitis) doesn't affect the lungs directly, but it often causes coughing because mucus from the sinuses drips down the throat into the lungs, irritating them. This is particularly a problem at night.

Home Treatment of Cough

The mucus in the bronchial tubes may be made thinner and less sticky by several means. Increasing the humidity in the air will help; a vaporizer and a steamy shower are two ways to add humidity. Drinking a lot of fluids is helpful, particularly if a fever has dehydrated the body. Glyceryl guaiacolate (Robitussin) may help liquefy mucus so it can be coughed out of the lungs more easily. Decongestants (Sudafed) and/or antihistamines (Benadryl) may help if the cough is caused by nasal or sinus material dripping down into the lungs. (Note: These medicines should otherwise be avoided because they dry the mucus and make it thicker. Over-the-counter cold medicines almost always contain antihistamine—and/or decongestant and/or expectorant—in some combination.)

Dry, tickling coughs are often relieved by sucking on cough lozenges or hard candy. Dextromethorphan (Robitussin-DM) is an effective cough suppressant that you can buy without a prescription, but neither this nor codeine (available only with a prescription) will completely get rid of a cough, even at a high dosage.

DIARRHEA

Many of the concerns with diarrhea are the same as those with nausea and vomiting (see page 124). Dehydration is the greatest risk and can require intravenous medicines when it is severe. Diarrhea that is jet-black or bloody may indicate bleeding from the intestines. Most people with diarrhea will have cramping and intermittent gas-like pains, but severe, steady abdominal pain could be more serious.

In people with HIV/AIDS, diarrhea can be caused by viral, bacterial, or parasitic infections and is often caused by the effect of HIV itself on the intestines. In many cases, it is a side effect of a drug. Several anti-HIV medicines can cause diarrhea, including nelfinavir (Viracept), ritonavir (Norvir), amprenavir (Agenerase), didanosine (ddI, Videx), and others. Antibiotics and anticancer drugs also cause diarrhea in some people. If medications seem to be responsible for diarrhea, it is important to discuss this with your doctor.

Home Treatment of Diarrhea

Home treatment of diarrhea is directed at getting enough fluid into the body to prevent dehydration. Sip clear fluids, such as water or ginger ale. If you are vomiting and nothing will stay down, suck on ice chips; this is usually tolerated and provides fluid. Gatorade, bouillon, and Jell-O are also good sources of liquid. The next step is to move on to constipating foods; follow the "BRAT" rule: bananas, rice, applesauce, and toast. Dairy foods and fats will not absorb well and should be avoided for a few days.

DIARRHEA ACTION CHART

Is either of the following present?   Yes   See doctor
• *Black or bloody stools*   →
• *Severe, steady abdominal pain*

now.

No ↓

Do you have any signs of dehydration?   Yes   See doctor
• *Extreme thirst*   →
• *Very dry mouth*
• *Dark urine*
• *Lightheadedness*

today.

No ↓

Are you taking *antibiotics*?   Yes   Call doctor.

No ↓   →

Has *diarrhea* been severe for longer   Yes   Call doctor.
than 5 days without improvement?   →

No ↓

Home treatment (see page 118)

Nonprescription remedies such as Kaopectate will make the stool more solid, but they won't change the amount or frequency of the stools. Many cases of diarrhea will get better on their own within five days, but if this doesn't happen, you should call your doctor. You may eventually need stronger medication to slow down the intestinal tract.

FEVER

The most common cause of fevers in HIV/AIDS is infection. The single most common cause of fever is probably HIV itself. Fever can be caused by viral, bacterial, and parasitic infections, and is sometimes caused by cancers or medications. Fever is a distressing symptom, although it's rarely dangerous in itself. However, the infection that might be causing the fever could be very serious. Everyone needs to know how to measure a fever and how to decide when it's time to see the doctor.

If you have HIV, you should have a thermometer and know how to use it properly. Both Fahrenheit and centigrade thermometers are okay. If your temperature is greater than or equal to 101°F, it is important to consider whether you could have one of the serious, emergency AIDS-associated infections. These include meningitis, an infection of the lining of the brain that causes *neck stiffness* and *confusion*, and *Pneumocystis* pneumonia (PCP), an infection of the lungs that causes *dry cough* and *shortness of breath*, particularly upon exertion. People with a permanent central intravenous line (usually inserted into the upper arm or the chest) are at risk for bacterial sepsis (blood poisoning) and should be evaluated promptly upon developing new fevers.

If none of these problems is present, the fever could still be serious but probably doesn't require immediate attention by a doctor. The important consideration is what symptoms are associated with the fever and how they should be managed.

Home Treatment of Fever

There are two ways to reduce a fever: sponging and medication. Sponging the skin with tepid water will bring the body temperature down as the water evaporates. Medications to lower fever include aspirin, acetaminophen (Tylenol, Datril), and ibuprofen (Motrin, Advil). Adults can take two aspirins every three to four hours as required. Acetamenophen is taken similarly and is often confused with aspirin, but it is a completely different medicine. It has the same temperature-lowering effect as aspirin but causes less stomach upset. On the other hand, acetaminophen can cause liver damage in high doses, and overdose can be fatal. Because aspirin and acetaminophen

FEVER ACTION CHART

Is your temperature greater than or equal to 101°F (38.3°C) and associated with
• *Neck stiffness?*
• *Lethargy or confusion?*
• *Seizure?*
• *Severe irritability?*

Yes → See doctor now.

No ↓

Is your temperature greater than or equal to 101°F (38.3°C) and associated with *dry cough and severe shortness of breath?*

Yes → See doctor now.

No ↓

Is this a *new fever*, and are you using a central IV (intravenous) line for medications?

Yes → Call or see doctor today.

No ↓

Is the *fever* associated with a new *skin rash* or *skin sores?*

Yes → Call or see doctor today.

No ↓

Is the *fever* associated with
• *Headache?*
• *Sore throat?*
• *Cough* (not short of breath)
• *Diarrhea?*
• *Urinary problems?*

Yes → See section on the associated problem.

No ↓

Home Treatment (page XXX)

are different drugs, they can be given together to control fever when one or the other alone is not effective. When you do this, stagger the doses every three hours, alternating doses of aspirin and acetaminophen.

HEADACHE

Headache is the single most frequent complaint of modern times. The most common causes of headache are tension (something that people with HIV/AIDS often have) and muscle spasms. Medications can also lead to headaches; zidovudine (AZT) is a frequent cause for some people.

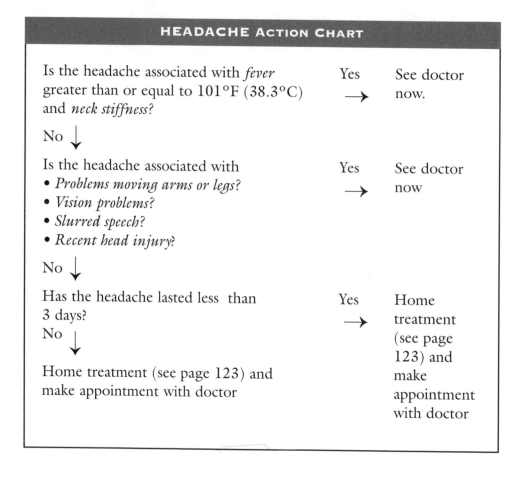

HEADACHE Action Chart

Is the headache associated with *fever* greater than or equal to 101°F (38.3°C) and *neck stiffness?*   Yes → See doctor now.

No ↓

Is the headache associated with   Yes → See doctor now
• *Problems moving arms or legs?*
• *Vision problems?*
• *Slurred speech?*
• *Recent head injury?*

No ↓

Has the headache lasted less than 3 days?   Yes → Home treatment (see page 123) and make appointment with doctor

No ↓

Home treatment (see page 123) and make appointment with doctor

However, there are several opportunistic diseases that can start out as headaches in people with HIV/ AIDS. Headache associated with *fever* and a *neck so stiff that the chin cannot be touched to the chest* suggests the possibility of meningitis, a serious infection of the lining of the brain. Headaches could be caused by infection or a tumor in the brain itself if they are associated with neurological problems such as *slurred speech, weakness or paralysis in the arms or legs*, or new *visual problems*. Any headache that comes after a *severe head injury* could be serious.

Home Treatment of Headache

The usual over-the-counter drugs (aspirin, acetaminophen, ibuprofen) are quite effective in relieving headache. Headache also responds very well to techniques that help reduce stress and tension. Try massage or heat applied to the back of the upper neck, or simply resting with your eyes closed and your head supported. Meditation is often effective. Headaches that don't respond to these measures should be brought to the attention of a doctor.

IMPAIRED/DECREASED VISION

Your vision is important, so any vision change should lead you to see the doctor if it doesn't improve on its own. The most common causes of vision problems in people with HIV/AIDS are no different than in other people: nearsightedness and farsightedness. Vision will also sometimes be affected by medications, high blood sugar, headaches, eye strain, or fatigue. When one of these things is causing vision problems, the change is usually gradual and about equal in both eyes. You should see a doctor, although this isn't an emergency. But HIV/AIDS can also lead to CMV (cytomegalovirus) retinitis, an infection of the back of the eye that can damage the visual field severely. In its worst forms, CMV retinitis can lead to blindness, but it can be arrested with medications. This is why you should see your doctor for any visual change, and see him or her *promptly* about a rapid or asymmetric visual change.

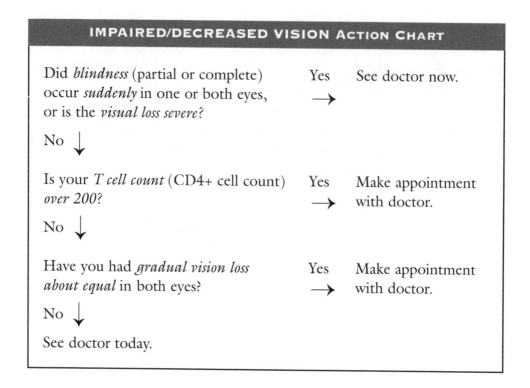

IMPAIRED/DECREASED VISION ACTION CHART

Did *blindness* (partial or complete) occur *suddenly* in one or both eyes, or is the *visual loss severe?* — Yes → See doctor now.

No ↓

Is your *T cell count* (CD4+ cell count) *over 200?* — Yes → Make appointment with doctor.

No ↓

Have you had *gradual vision loss about equal* in both eyes? — Yes → Make appointment with doctor.

No ↓

See doctor today.

Home Treatment of Impaired/Decreased Vision

If you experience temporary changes in vision caused by medications or fatigue, try resting with your eyes closed in a darkened room for a few minutes. On bright days, be sure to protect your eyes with sunglasses; this will decrease strain and allow your eyes to accommodate more easily. Permanent changes in your vision should be discussed with your doctor.

NAUSEA AND VOMITING

Many of the concerns with nausea and vomiting are the same as those with diarrhea (see page 118). Medications are the most common cause of nausea in people with HIV/AIDS, although viral infections can also cause problems. *Dehydration* is the greatest risk; as with diarrhea, intravenous medicines may be needed when it gets severe. People with severe dehydration often experience *dizziness, severe thirst, dry mouth and tongue,*

NAUSEA AND VOMITING Action Chart

Are any of the following present? Yes See doctor
- *Black or bloody vomit* → now.
- *Severe, steady abdominal pain*
- *Headache and stiff neck*

No ↓

Do you have any signs of dehydration? Yes See doctor
- *Extreme thirst* → now.
- *Very dry mouth*
- *Dark urine*
- *Lightheadedness*

No ↓

Did this begin after starting a *new* Yes Call doctor.
medication? →

No ↓

Are you *pregnant*, or do you think Yes Call doctor.
you might be pregnant? →

No ↓

Have you been *vomiting* for more than Yes Call doctor.
3 days without improvement? →

No ↓

Home treatment (see page 126)

decreased amounts of urine, dark urine, and *wrinkled, dry skin. Vomit that is bloody or black* may indicate that severe intestinal bleeding is present. This problem is particularly bad in people with liver disease. An infection of the brain can sometimes lead to nausea and vomiting, so if you have a *headache* and a *stiff neck*, see your doctor right away. Women who are sexually active should always consider the possibility that their nausea is due to pregnancy. The best way to know for sure is to get a pregnancy test, either over the counter at your local drugstore or in your doctor's office.

Many medications used in HIV/AIDS care can cause nausea. The anti-HIV drugs that can cause stomach upset include zidovidune (AZT, Retrovir), didanosine (ddI, Videx), lamivudine (3TC, Epivir), nelfinavir (Viracept), ritonavir (Norvir), and amprenavir (Agenerase); but in truth, many different medications can have this side effect. Antibiotics and anti-cancer drugs are other examples. If nausea begins soon after you start a new medicine, call the doctor.

Home Treatment of Nausea and Vomiting

The goal of home treatment of nausea is to get as much fluid as possible into your body without further upsetting your stomach. Sip clear fluids, such as water or ginger ale. Suck on ice chips if nothing else will stay down. Don't drink too much at any one time, as this will aggravate the stomach. Add Gatorade, bouillon, soups, and Jell-O as your condition improves. If the vomiting does not go away within three days, call the doctor.

SHORTNESS OF BREATH

Shortness of breath is normal during strenuous activity. But if you get "winded" at rest or with only minimal exertion, or if you wake up at night short of breath, you have a serious symptom that should be evaluated promptly by a doctor. In people with HIV/AIDS, the major concern is pneumonia, most often caused by *Pneumocystis* pneumonia (PCP). PCP almost always causes a dry cough and a fever, so these symptoms are very important.

SHORTNESS OF BREATH ACTION CHART		
Do you have *shortness of breath at rest*, or with *minimal exertion*? No ↓	Yes →	See doctor now.
Is the shortness of breath associated with *dry cough* and *fever*? No ↓	Yes →	See doctor now.
Home treatment (see Chapter 9) and make appointment with doctor.		

There are several other causes of chronic shortness of breath, including lung damage caused by previous lung infections, anemia, and smoking-induced lung disease.

Home Treatment of Shortness of Breath

Several suggestions that are often helpful for people with shortness of breath are given in Chapter 9, "Understanding the Symptom Cycle."

SORE THROAT

A sore throat is almost never a life-threatening problem, but it can be painful. Sore throats can be caused by several infections. "Cold" viruses are the most common cause and cannot be treated successfully with antibiotics; they must be allowed to run their course. Mononucleosis ("mono") is a viral infection that causes a more severe, prolonged illness with painful swelling and soreness in the throat. Even though it sounds formidable, mono rarely causes complications and usually gets better with rest. As is the case with colds, antibiotics won't combat the symptoms of mononucleosis.

Streptococcal bacteria ("strep throat") are another common cause of sore throat. Strep throat should be treated with antibiotics in order to prevent the small chance of an abscess forming and to prevent the kidney damage that can sometimes occur. It's hard to tell when a sore throat might be strep throat, but it's unlikely when the sore throat is a minor part of a typical cold (runny nose, stuffy ears, etc.). A high temperature, pus in the back of the throat, or swollen tonsils can be clues indicating that strep throat may be present. Sore throat in people with HIV/AIDS can also be caused by infection with candida (thrush) or by ulcers in the throat from herpes or CMV (cytomegalovirus) infections.

SORE THROAT ACTION CHART

Do you have *severe difficulty swallowing* or *difficulty breathing?*

Yes → See doctor now.

No ↓

Are either of the following conditions present?
• *Temperature of 101°F or more*
• *Pus in the back of the throat*

Yes → Call the doctor today.

No ↓

Are your *tonsils swollen?*

Yes → Obtain a throat culture.

No ↓

Has your sore throat *lasted longer than 10 days?*

Yes → Call the doctor today.

No ↓

Home treatment (see page 129)

None of these conditions is an emergency (unless, of course, you are unable to eat or breathe), but a sore throat should sometimes be looked at by a doctor. If your sore throat doesn't seem to be associated with usual cold symptoms or if it lasts longer than ten days, you should contact your doctor.

Home Treatment of Sore Throat

Cold liquids, aspirin, ibuprofen, and acetaminophen are effective for the pain and fever associated with some sore throats. If you have had oral thrush in the past and think you might have it now (white, cottage cheese-like material in your mouth), you should start the thrush medicine your doctor gave you (usually clotrimazole (Mycelex) "troches"). Home remedies that may help include saltwater gargles and honey or lemon in tea.

Urination Problems: Painful, Frequent, or Bloody Urination

Urinary infections are much more common in women than in men, but men can get them too, especially if they have HIV/AIDS. The most common symptoms of urinary infection are *pain or burning on urination, frequent urgent urination*, and *blood in the urine*. But sometimes these symptoms are not caused by infection. They can also be due to excessive use of caffeine-containing beverages (coffee, tea, or cola), bladder spasms, or even anxiety. Bladder infection in women is often caused by sexual activity.

If *fever, vomiting, back pain*, or *teeth-chattering or body-shaking chills* are present, this suggests that the infection may have spread from the bladder to the kidneys and may be much more serious. Bladder infections are common during pregnancy, when the treatment is more difficult. For women who get repeated bladder infections, it is important to remember to wipe the toilet tissue from front to back after urinating. Most bacteria that cause bladder infections come from the rectum.

```
┌─────────────────────────────────────────────────────────────┐
│          URINATION PROBLEMS ACTION CHART                    │
├─────────────────────────────────────────────────────────────┤
```

URINATION PROBLEMS ACTION CHART

Are the symptoms (painful, frequent, or bloody urination) associated with fever, vomiting, back pain, or shaking chills, or is there a chance you could be *pregnant*?

Yes ⟶ See doctor today.

No ↓

Is the problem associated with a new, irritating *vaginal discharge*?

Yes ⟶ See doctor today.

No ↓

Is the vaginal discharge associated with pain in the abdomen?

Yes ⟶ See doctor today.

No ↓

Home treatment (see below) and call the doctor today.

Home Treatment of Urination Problems

Home treatment involves drinking a lot of fluids. Drink as much as several gallons of fluid in the first twenty-four hours after symptoms start. Bacteria are literally washed out of the body with the resulting urination. Drink fruit juices to put more acid into the urine. Begin home treatment as soon as you notice the symptoms. Relief may well begin before you see the doctor.

Irritation from the vagina can sometimes cause frequent urination or blood in the urine. When this happens, the infection may not be in the urinary system, but in the vagina or cervix. If there is *pain in the abdomen* along with vaginal discharge, this suggests a potentially serious disease, ranging from gonorrhea to an ectopic pregnancy in the fallopian tube.

These conditions are also suggested by *bloody discharge that comes between periods, frequently or in large amounts.* All these conditions should be evaluated by the doctor. Candida yeast (the same thing that causes thrush) often causes *discharge from the vagina—it looks like white, cheesy material.* It may respond to over-the-counter anti-yeast medications (Monistat, Mycolog), but some women with HIV/AIDS need stronger medicines available only by prescription.

The major concern in women with discharge from the vagina is the possibility of sexually transmitted disease (STD). All the organisms that cause STDs can cause severe infections in women with HIV/AIDS. If sexual contact in the past few weeks may have led to an STD, you must see a doctor. It's okay to start home self-management, but make an appointment with the doctor, too.

Women who are taking antibiotics often get worse yeast infections in the vagina. To prevent these infections, it's helpful to eat yogurt, buttermilk, or sour cream and to use less sugar and drink less alcohol. It may be helpful to call the doctor for advice on changing medications.

SUGGESTED READING

Vickery, Donald M., and Fries, James F. *Take Care of Yourself.* 8th ed. Oxford: Perseus, 2004.

Ward, Darrell E. *The AmFAR AIDS Handbook: The Complete Guide to Understanding HIV and AIDS.* New York: W.W. Norton & Company, 1998.

CHAPTER NINE

Understanding the Symptom Cycle

Being able to identify and evaluate symptoms is only part of what is necessary to become an effective self-manager. The other part is being able to understand the different causes of these symptoms, so that you can prevent them or manage them better. Although it may seem as though it should be easy to identify symptoms and what their causes are, this is not always so. People with HIV/AIDS experience many symptoms, including fatigue, stress, anger, depression, and sleeping problems. Often these symptoms are complex and interrelated, creating a vicious cycle in which one symptom feeds into another, causing more discomfort and other problems. Sometimes the symptoms and associated problems are not easily treated with medications, so it is necessary to find other ways to deal with them.

In this chapter we discuss some of the more common symptoms that people with HIV/AIDS experience. We look at the different factors that cause or intensify these symptoms and suggest some ways to break the cycle.

ANGER—WHY ME?

Anger is one of the most common responses to having HIV/AIDS. The uncertainty and unpredictability of living with HIV/AIDS threatens what you have fought all your life to achieve—independence and control. The loss of control over your body and loss of independence in life create feelings of frustration, helplessness, and hopelessness, all of which fuel the anger. In fact, at various times during the course of your illness, you may find yourself asking, "Why me?" You may wonder what you did to deserve this. All of these are normal responses to HIV/AIDS.

You may be angry with yourself, your partner, family, friends, health care providers, God, or the world in general—for a variety of reasons. You may be angry at yourself for becoming HIV infected in the first place. You may be angry at your partner, family, and friends because they don't do things the way you would like them done. You may be angry at your doctor because he or she cannot "fix" you. Other people's attitudes about you and this disease may also anger you. Sometimes your anger may be misplaced, as when you find yourself yelling at the cat or dog. Misplaced anger is quite common, especially if you are not even aware that you are angry or why.

Sometimes the anger is not just a response to having HIV/AIDS but is actually the result of the disease process itself. For example, if you have suffered an infection that has affected a certain part of the brain, your ability to express or suppress emotions may be affected. Some people who have had brain infections thus cry "for no reason" or have flares of temper.

Recognizing (or admitting) that you are angry and identifying why, or with whom, are important in learning how to manage your anger. This task also involves finding constructive ways to express your anger. If not expressed, the anger becomes unhealthy. It can build up until it becomes explosive and offends others or is turned inward, intensifying other disease symptoms, such as depression.

Dealing with Anger

There are several things that you can do to help manage your anger:

- *Learn how to communicate your anger verbally*, preferably without blaming or offending others. (Using "I" messages rather than "you" messages to express your feelings will help you avoid blaming; these are discussed more fully in Chapter 14, "Communicating.") However, if you choose to express your anger verbally, know that many people will not be able to help you. Most of us are not very good at, or comfortable with, dealing with angry people, even if the anger is justified.

Therefore, you may also find it useful to seek counseling or join a support group. Voluntary organizations, such as your local AIDS foundation, may have information about these.

- *Modify your expectations.* You have done this throughout your life. For example, as a child you thought you could become anything—a firefighter, a ballet dancer, a doctor. As you grew older, however, you reevaluated these expectations along with your talents and interests. From this reevaluation, you modified your plans. You can use this same process to deal with the effects of HIV/AIDS on your life. For example, it may be unrealistic to expect that you will get "all better" and no longer need treatment. However, it is realistic to expect that you can still do many pleasurable things. You have the ability to affect the progress of your illness by slowing it down or preventing it from becoming worse. Changing your expectations can help you change your perspective. Instead of dwelling on the ten percent of things you can no longer do, think about the ninety percent of things you still can do. You may even be able to find new activities or hobbies to replace the old ones. Learning to think positively or talk to yourself positively can also help to change your perspective.

- *Channel your anger through new activities,* such as exercise, writing, listening to music, and painting. Some people find these to be excellent outlets for angry feelings.

In short, anger is a normal response to having HIV/AIDS. Part of learning to manage the disease involves acknowledging this anger and finding constructive ways to deal with it.

DEPRESSION

Depression can be a frightening word. Some people prefer to say that they are "blue" or "feeling down." Whatever you call it, depression is a normal reaction to HIV/AIDS. It is not always easy to recognize when you are depressed. Even more difficult is recognizing when you may be becoming depressed and then catching yourself before you fall into a deep depression. Just as there are many degrees of pain, there are many degrees of depression. If your disease is a significant problem in your life, you almost certainly have, or have had, some problems with depression. Although depression is felt by everyone at some time, it is how you handle it that makes the difference. There are many different signs of depression, which will be discussed later in this section.

Emotions Leading to Depression

Several emotions can lead to depression:

- *Fear, anxiety, and/or uncertainty about the future.* Whether these feelings result from worries about finances, the disease process, your partner, or your family, constant worry about these issues can lead to depression if they are not addressed by you and those involved. In Chapter 16, "Planning for Now—and the Future," we discuss some decisions that all of us will have to make at some time in our lives. By confronting these issues early on, you will put your mind at rest and have more time to enjoy life.

- *Frustration.* A number of things can call up feelings of frustration. You may find yourself thinking, "I just can't do what I want," "I feel so helpless," "I used to be able to do this myself," or "Why doesn't anyone understand me?" Feelings like these can leave you feeling more alone and isolated, the longer you hold on to them.

- *Loss of control over your life.* Whether it comes from having to rely on medications, having to see a doctor on a regular basis, or having to count on others to help you perform your daily activities—such as bathing, dressing, and preparing meals—the feeling of losing control can make you lose faith in yourself and your abilities. Your life has suddenly become a team sport in which you are no longer the coach. You are now a player with someone else calling the plays.

Although the signs of depression are listed separately, they are often experienced in combination, making it more difficult to determine what is really at the root of the depression. Also, we often do not recognize when we are depressed or do not wish to admit to ourselves that we are actually depressed. Learning to recognize the signs of depression is the first step in learning how to manage it.

Dealing with Depression

It is undeniable that having HIV/AIDS can be very depressing. We would not try to tell you that you should not have feelings of depression about your illness. However, just as the *physical* deconditioning resulting from HIV/AIDS can make you feel weak and helpless, leading to less physical activity and even more deconditioning, depression can lead to a vicious cycle of *emotional* "deconditioning." (See Figure 1.1, p. 6.) Depression can cause you to feel helpless and hopeless and to let go of many of your normally pleasurable activities, which in turn makes life seem even more bleak.

Depression makes us see things darkly, and to tend to believe that nothing can be changed. Not so! Depression is something that you *can* manage, just like any other symptom of HIV/AIDS. As part of being very depressed, however, you may not be able to muster the strength to get started. You may need to force yourself into action or get someone to help you do the things that will help.

Here are some active steps you can take to manage depression:

- *Seek help immediately if you feel like hurting yourself or someone else.* Call your mental health center, doctor, suicide prevention center, a friend, spiritual counselor, or community center. Do not delay. Do it now. Often, just talking with an understanding person or health professional will be enough to help you through this mood.

- *If you can, stop taking tranquilizers or narcotic painkillers,* such as Valium, Librium, codeine, Vicodin, sleeping medications, or other "downers" if you use them. Some people do need to take these sorts of medicines, so you should discuss any medication change you make with your doctor. These drugs can intensify depression, so if you can stop taking them, you're likely to be better off. Your depression may be a drug side effect. If you are not sure what you are taking or are uncertain whether what you're experiencing is a side effect, check with a doctor or

SIGNS OF DEPRESSION

- *Loss of interest in friends or activities.* Not wanting to talk to anyone or answer the phone or doorbell.

- *Difficulty sleeping,* changed sleeping patterns, interrupted sleep, or sleeping more than usual. You may go to sleep easily but awaken often and be unable to go back to sleep.

- *Changes in eating habits.* This may range from a loss of interest in food to unusually erratic or excessive eating.

- *Unintentional weight change,* either gain or loss, of more than 10 pounds in a short period of time.

- *Loss of interest in personal care and grooming.*

- *A general feeling of unhappiness* lasting longer than 6 weeks.

- *Loss of interest in being held or in sex.* These problems can sometimes be caused by medication side effects, so it is important that you talk them over with your doctor.

- *Suicidal thoughts.* If your unhappiness has caused you to think about killing yourself, get help from your doctor, good friends, a member of the clergy, a psychologist, or a social worker. These feelings will pass and you will feel better, so get help and don't let a tragedy happen to you and your loved ones.

- *Frequent accidents.* Watch for a pattern of increased carelessness, accidents while walking or driving, dropping things, and so forth. Of course you must take into account how much the physical problems caused by your disease, such as unsteady balance or slowed reaction time, may be contributing to these incidents.

- *Poor self-image or low self-esteem.* A feeling of worthlessness, a negative image of your body, wondering, "Is it all worth it?"

- *Frequent arguments.* A tendency to blow up easily over minor matters, things that never bothered you before.

- *Loss of energy.* Feeling tired all the time.

- *Inability to make decisions.* Feeling confused and unable to concentrate.

pharmacist. Before discontinuing a prescription medication, *always* check—at least by phone—with the prescribing physician. There may be important reasons to keep taking the medicine, or there may be withdrawal reactions.

- *Cut back on alcohol.* Although you may be drinking to feel better, alcohol is also a downer. There is virtually no way to escape depression unless you cleanse your brain of chemical downers such as alcohol. For most people, one or two drinks in the evening is not a problem, but if your mind is not free of alcohol during most of the day, you are having trouble with this drug.

- *Continue your daily activities.* Get dressed every day, make your bed, get out of the house, go shopping, walk your dog. Plan and cook meals. Force yourself to do these things even if you don't feel like it.

- *Visit with friends.* Call them on the phone. Plan to go to the movies or on other outings. Do it!

- *Join a group.* Get involved in a church group, a discussion group, a community college class, a self-help class, or a nutrition program.

- *Volunteer.* People who help other people are seldom depressed.

- *Make plans and carry them out.* Look to the future. Plant some young trees. Look forward to some special occasion. If you know that one time of the year is especially difficult, such as Christmas or a birthday, make specific plans for that period. Don't wait to see what happens. Be prepared.

- *Don't move to a new setting* without first visiting for a few weeks. Moving can be a sign of withdrawal, and depression often intensifies when you are in a location away from friends and acquaintances. Your troubles usually move with you.

- *Take a vacation* with relatives or friends. Vacations can be as simple as a few days in a nearby city or in a resort just a few miles down the road. Rather than go alone, look into trips sponsored by colleges, your city recreation department, the "Y," clubs, support groups, or church groups.

- *Participate in twenty to thirty minutes of physical exercise every day.*

- *Make a list of self-rewards.* You can reward yourself by doing something special for yourself, such as reading at a set time or seeing a play. Anything, big or small, that you can look forward to during the day can help combat feelings of depression.

- *If you are very depressed, talk to your doctor or nurse about taking an antidepressant medication.* Such drugs can be very helpful, and one of them may be appropriate for you.

Depression feeds on depression, so break the cycle. The success of your self-management program depends on it. Depression may also interfere with your treatment. It may keep you from taking your medication or make you eat poorly but depression is not permanent, and you can hasten its disappearance. Focus on your pride, your friends, your goals, and your positive surroundings. How you respond to depression is a self-fulfilling prophecy. When you believe that things will get better, they will.

FATIGUE

HIV/AIDS can drain your energy. For many people, fatigue is a very real problem and not "all in the mind." It can keep you from doing the things you'd like to do. Furthermore, the effects of fatigue may be misunderstood or underestimated by others. Sometimes family, friends, and partners do not understand the unpredictability of the fatigue associated with HIV/AIDS and may misinterpret it as a lack of interest in certain activities or a desire to be alone.

Common Causes of Fatigue

Fatigue can have many causes, including these:

- *The disease itself.* When you have HIV/AIDS, activities require more energy. The body is less efficient because some of the energy usually available for daily activities is now needed to help the body heal itself.

- *Inactivity.* Muscles that aren't used become deconditioned; that is, they become less efficient at doing what they are supposed to do. The heart, which is made of muscular tissue, can also become deconditioned. When this happens, the heart's ability to pump blood, nutrients, and oxygen to other parts of the body is decreased. When muscles do not receive the nutrients and oxygen they need to function properly, they tire more easily than muscles in good condition—the ones that receive an adequate supply of blood, oxygen, and nutrients through physical activity.

- *Poor nutrition.* Food is your basic source of energy. If the fuel you take in is not of top quality and/or in proper quantity, fatigue can result.

- *Insufficient rest.* For a variety of reasons, there will be times when you do not get enough sleep or have poor-quality sleep. This can also result in fatigue. The final section of this chapter deals with sleep problems.

- *Emotions.* Stress and depression can also cause fatigue. Most people are aware of the connection between stress and feeling tired, but fatigue is also an important symptom of depression.

If fatigue is a problem for you, your first job is to determine the cause.

- Are you *exercising*?

- Are you *eating well*?

- Are you getting enough good-quality *sleep*?

If you answer "no" to any of these questions, you may be well on the way to determining the reasons for your fatigue. The important thing to remember about your fatigue is that it may be caused by many things other than your illness. Therefore, in order to fight and prevent fatigue, you must address the cause(s).

Dealing with Fatigue

People often say they can't exercise because they feel fatigued. This creates a negative cycle: You are fatigued because of a lack of exercise, and then you don't exercise because of the fatigue. Believe it or not, if this is your problem, motivating yourself to do a little exercise next time you are fatigued may be the answer. You don't have to run a marathon; just go outdoors and take a short walk. If this is not possible, then walk around your house. See Chapter 11, "Exercising for Fun and Fitness," for more information on getting started on an exercise program.

If your fatigue is caused by eating too many empty calories in the form of junk food or alcohol, the solution is to eat higher-quality food, in proper quantity. For some people, the problem may be a decreased interest in food, leading to subsequent weight loss. Other people may not absorb food well because of gastrointestinal (GI) tract problems. Chapter 12, "Healthy Eating," and Chapter 13, "Food Safety and Preparation Tips," discuss in greater detail some of the problems associated with eating poorly and offer advice for improving your eating habits.

If you are having trouble getting to sleep, getting enough sleep, or staying asleep during the night, then it is very likely that your body is not getting the rest it needs to replenish its energy. This can lead to fatigue. We offer some suggestions to help you get a better night's sleep later in this chapter.

If emotions are causing your fatigue, rest will not help; in fact, it may make you feel worse. Fatigue is often a sign of depression, and we discussed ways to deal with depression earlier in this chapter. Stress can also cause fatigue; at the end of this chapter, we suggest ways to manage it.

PAIN

Pain is a problem shared by many people with HIV/AIDS. In fact, it may be their number one concern. As with most symptoms, pain can have many causes.

Common Causes of Pain

The four most common causes of pain are the following:

- *The disease itself.* Pain can come from damaged nerves, swollen internal organs, or irritated skin, just to name a few.

- *Tense muscles.* When something hurts, the muscles in that area become tense. This is your body's natural reaction to pain.

- *Muscle deconditioning.* It is common for people with HIV/AIDS to become less active, leading to a weakening of the muscles, or muscle deconditioning. When a muscle is weak, it tends to complain any time it is used. Thus, even the slightest activity can sometimes lead to pain and stiffness.

- *Fear and depression.* When you are afraid, frustrated, or depressed, everything, including pain, seems worse. This is not to imply that the pain is not real. Rather, fear and depression tend to heighten sensations and make an already bad experience worse.

Because pain comes from many sources, pain management must be aimed at all of those that apply. Medications can help with some disease-caused pain; for example, they can help open blood vessels and bronchial tubes or reduce pain caused by inflammation.

Dealing with Pain

Two of the best ways of dealing with pain are exercise and cognitive pain-management techniques, such as relaxation and visualization, in which you actively use your mind to help manage your symptoms. The benefits of exercise, and tips for starting an exercise program, are discussed in Chapter 11; using your mind to manage symptoms is discussed in Chapter 10.

In addition to exercise and cognitive pain management, several other techniques—such as heat, cold, and massage—are sometimes useful for localized pain. These three methods work by stimulating the skin and other tissues surrounding the painful area, which increases the blood flow to the area.

- *Heat.* You can stimulate the blood flow by applying a heating pad or by taking a warm bath or shower (with the water flow directed at the painful area). Limit the application to fifteen or twenty minutes at a time.

- *Cold.* Some people prefer cold for soothing the pain. A bag of frozen peas or corn makes an inexpensive, reusable cold pack. Limit the application to fifteen or twenty minutes at a time.

- *Massage* is actually one of the oldest forms of pain management. Hippocrates (ca. 460–380 B.C.) said, "physicians must be experienced in many things, but assuredly also in the rubbing that can bind a joint that is loose and loosen a joint that is too hard." Self-massage is a simple method that you can use with little practice or preparation. It stimulates the skin, underlying tissues, and muscles by means of applying pressure. Some people like to use a mentholated cream with self-massage because it gives a cooling effect. Massage, however, is not appropriate for all cases of pain. Do not use self-massage for a "hot joint" (one that is red, swollen, and hot to the touch) or an infected area, or if you are suffering from phlebitis, thrombophlebitis, or skin eruptions. For more details on specific types of massage, see the "Suggested Reading" list at the end of this chapter.

SHORTNESS OF BREATH

Shortness of breath can be a chronic symptom, or it can be caused by an acute infection that could be dangerous if not cleared up with proper treatment. To rule out the possibility of an acute infection, be sure to check your symptoms against the Shortness of Breath action chart in Chapter 8, "Evaluating Common Symptoms of HIV/AIDS," before going on to the things discussed in this section. Shortness of breath, like fatigue and stress, can have many causes. But whatever the cause, shortness of breath indicates that your body is not getting the oxygen that it needs.

Common Causes of Shortness of Breath

Here are some of the most common physiological changes that take place as a result of HIV/AIDS and that lead to shortness of breath:

- *Damage to the air sacs in the lungs,* possibly resulting from some lung infections. Such damage causes the lungs to be less efficient at getting oxygen into the blood and carbon dioxide out. Although the body can adjust to this change to some extent, when there is a sudden change in your "normal" breathing pattern (for example, when you walk up stairs quickly) the lungs cannot always keep up.

- *Narrowing of the airways to the air sacs and excess mucus production.* Because the airways have narrowed, there is less room for air to flow through to get to the lungs. Excess mucus production also decreases the amount of space available for oxygen to get to the lungs. These changes occur with both asthma and chronic bronchitis.

- *Anemia.* Oxygen is carried in the red blood cells, so people who are anemic (have too few red blood cells) may develop shortness of breath.

- *Deconditioning of muscles.* The deconditioning process can affect the breathing muscles or any of the other muscles in your body. When muscles become deconditioned, they are less efficient in doing what they are supposed to do, so they require more energy (and oxygen) to perform their activities. In the case of the breathing muscles, the process of clearing the lungs becomes less efficient, and less space is left for fresh air to be inhaled.

- *Anxiety and stress.* Anxiety can speed up your breathing and make it difficult to take full, deep breaths.

Dealing with Shortness of Breath

Just as there are many causes of shortness of breath, there are many things you can do to manage this problem.

- *Don't stop what you are doing or hurry up to finish* when you feel short of breath. Instead, slow down. If shortness of breath continues, stop for a few minutes. If you are still short of breath, take medication if it has been prescribed by your doctor. Often shortness of breath is frightening, and this fear can cause two additional problems. First, fear can cause the body to release hormones that may cause more shortness of breath. Second, fear may cause you to stop your activity and thus never build up the endurance necessary to help your breathing. The basic rule is to take things slowly and in steps.

- *Increase your activity level gradually,* generally by not more than twenty-five percent each week. Thus, if you are now able to garden comfortably for twenty minutes, next week increase your time by a maximum of five minutes. Once you can garden comfortably for twenty-five minutes, you can again add a few more minutes.

- *Don't smoke.* If you are a smoker, this is easier said than done. Most smokers are addicted to smoking and nicotine without realizing it. When you try to quit, the unpleasant symptoms of withdrawal—such as lightheadedness, sleepiness, and headaches—make it very difficult. These symptoms subside in a few weeks but can still leave you with a craving for nicotine. A nicotine patch or gum can help you through the process of withdrawal. Another alternative is to find ways to distract or occupy yourself until the urge to smoke passes, such as chewing gum, walking around for a few minutes, brushing your teeth, or calling a friend. With time, the urges become less frequent.

  In addition to getting over the addiction to nicotine, you may find that you miss the physical motions associated with smoking. Try to find something else to keep your hands busy. You may also need to distract yourself or learn to substitute another activity for smoking when you are drinking coffee, finishing meals, reading, or watching television.

  It is the fear of failing that keeps some from even trying to quit. Whatever your reasons or difficulties are, however, there are many resources that can help you when you decide to quit, such as the American Cancer Society, the American Heart Association, the American Lung Association, your local community hospital or health maintenance organization, and the public health department. Many of these organizations offer courses or materials to help you stop smoking on your own or in a group setting.

- *Avoid the smoke of others.* Avoiding "secondhand smoke" is as important in managing shortness of breath as stopping smoking. This may sometimes be hard to do because friends who smoke do not realize how difficult they are making your life. Your job is to tell them. Explain that their smoke is causing breathing problems for you, and you would appreciate it if they would not smoke when you are around. Make your house a "No Smoking" zone. Ask people to smoke outside.

- *Use your medications and oxygen as prescribed by your doctor.* We are constantly bombarded with messages that drugs are bad and not to be used. In many cases, this is correct. However, when you have a chronic disease, drugs can be lifesavers. Don't try to skimp, cut down, or go without. At the same time, more is not "better," so don't take more than the prescribed dose of medications. Drugs, taken as prescribed, can make all the difference. This may mean using medications even when you are not having symptoms. It also means resisting the temptation to take more of the medication if the prescribed amount does not seem to be working. If you have questions about your medications or feel as if they are not working for you, discuss these concerns with your doctor before you stop taking the medication or start taking more than has been prescribed. Preventing a problem before it starts is much better than having to manage the problem later.

- *Drink plenty of fluids* if mucus is a problem, unless your doctor has advised you to restrict your fluid intake. The extra fluids will help to thin the mucus and make it easier to cough up. Using a humidifier may also be helpful.

- *Practice pursed-lip and diaphragmatic breathing.* As mentioned earlier, one of the problems that causes shortness of breath is a deconditioning of the diaphragm and breathing muscles. When this deconditioning occurs, the lungs are not able to empty properly, leaving less room for fresh air. Practiced together, pursed-lip and diaphragmatic breathing can help strengthen and improve the coordination and efficiency of the breathing muscles, and decrease the amount of energy needed to breathe. In addition, these two breathing exercises can be used with any of the techniques that use the power of your mind to manage your symptoms (often referred to as cognitive symptom management techniques and described in Chapter 10, "Using Your Mind to Manage Symptoms") or alone, to achieve a state of relaxation. See the accompanying tables for how-to advice on these breathing techniques.

PURSED-LIP BREATHING

Use this technique during exercise or any time you feel short of breath

1. Breathe in through your nose. This may be easier if you lean forward slightly.

2. Hold your breath briefly.

3. With your lips pursed as if you were going to whistle, breathe out slowly through your lips. Exhaling should take twice as long as inhaling.

4. Practice this technique for 5 to 10 minutes, two to four times a day.

DIAPHRAGMATIC BREATHING

Use this technique to strengthen your breathing muscles.

1. Lie on your back with pillows under your head and knees.

2. Place one hand on your stomach (at the base of your breastbone) and the other hand on your upper chest.

3. Inhale slowly through your nose, allowing your stomach to expand outward. Imagine that your lungs are filling with fresh air. The hand on your stomach should move upward, and the hand on your chest should not move.

4. Breathe out slowly, through pursed lips. At the same time, use your hand to gently push inward and upward on your abdomen.

5. Practice this technique for 10 to 15 minutes, three or four times a day, until it becomes automatic. If you begin to feel a little dizzy, rest.

SLEEPING PROBLEMS

While you are sleeping, the body can concentrate on healing because relatively little energy is required to maintain body functioning when we are asleep. When we do not get enough sleep, we may experience a variety of other symptoms, such as fatigue and lack of concentration. This does not mean that fatigue or lack of concentration is always caused by a lack of sleep; remember, the symptoms associated with HIV/AIDS can have many causes. However, if you have noticed a change in your sleep patterns, then the fatigue you are experiencing may, at least in part, be related to your problems with sleep.

Dealing with Sleep Problems

Many people feel powerless to solve their sleep problems, but there are many things you can do to help yourself get a good night's sleep. To sleep well, you need to: (1) have a good, comfortable place to sleep; (2) avoid putting substances in your body that interfere with sleep; (3) get into a sleep routine; and (4) learn to deal with things that may interrupt your sleep. Each of these items is covered below.

Before you even get into bed

- *Get a comfortable bed* that allows you to move around easily and provides good support. This usually means a good-quality, firm mattress that supports the spine and does not cause you to roll to the middle of the bed. A bed board, made of half- to three-quarter-inch plywood, can be placed between the mattress and the box spring to increase the firmness. Heated waterbeds or airbeds are helpful for some people because they support weight evenly by conforming to the body's shape. Other people find them to be very uncomfortable. If you are interested, try one out at a friend's home or a hotel for a few nights to decide whether it is right for you.

- *Elevate the head of your bed* on wooden blocks four to six inches thick to make breathing easier. You can get the same effect by using pillows that elevate your chest, shoulders, and head.

- *Keep the room at a comfortable, warm temperature.*

- *Use a vaporizer* if you live where the air is dry, and/or in cold weather, when your heating system lowers the humidity of the air in your house. Warm, moist air often makes breathing easier, leaving you with one less thing to worry about when trying to fall asleep.

- *Make your bedroom a place in which you feel safe and comfortable.* Keep a lamp and telephone by your bed within easy reach.

Things to avoid before bedtime

- *Avoid eating before bedtime.* Although you may feel sleepy after a big meal, eating is no way to help you fall asleep and get a good night's rest. Sleep is supposed to allow your body time to rest and recover; but when you eat, your body is kept busy with digestion, taking valuable time away from this healing process. Because going to sleep feeling hungry may also keep you awake, try drinking a glass of warm milk.

- *Avoid alcohol.* Contrary to the belief that alcohol will help you sleep better because it makes you feel more relaxed, alcohol actually disrupts your sleep cycle. Alcohol before bedtime can lead to shallow and fragmented sleep, and frequent awakenings throughout the night.

- *Avoid caffeine late in the day.* Because caffeine is a stimulant, it can keep you awake. Caffeine is found not only in coffee, but also in some types of teas, colas and other sodas, and chocolate.

- *Avoid eating foods with MSG (monosodium glutamate) late in the day.* Although Chinese foods are often singled out as containing MSG, many other types of food, especially prepackaged foods, may contain this food additive. Before purchasing a packaged meal, be sure to read the ingredient label to check that the food does not contain monosodium glutamate.

- *Don't smoke to help you sleep.* The nicotine in cigarettes is a stimulant. And aside from the fact that smoking itself can cause complications and worsening of lung problems, falling asleep with a lit cigarette is a fire hazard.

- *Don't take diet pills.* Diet pills often contain stimulants that may interfere with falling asleep and staying asleep.

- *Don't take sleeping pills.* Although sleeping pills sound like the perfect solution to sleep problems, they tend to become less effective over time. Also, many sleeping pills have a rebound effect—that is, if you stop taking them, it becomes more difficult to get to sleep. You may end up having even more problems than you had when you first started taking the sleeping pills. It is best to avoid using sleeping pills if at all possible.

Developing a routine

- *Set up a regular rest and sleep pattern.* Go to bed at the same time every night and get up at the same time every morning. If you wish to take a nap, take one in the afternoon, but do not take a nap after dinner. Stay awake until you are ready to go to bed.

- *Reset your sleep clock if your sleep pattern is way off the norm* (for example, if you go to bed at 4:00 A.M. and sleep until noon). To do so, try going to bed one hour earlier or later each day until you reach the hour you want to go to bed. This method may seem strange, but it seems to be the best way to reset your sleep clock.

- *Exercise at regular times each day.* Not only will the exercise help you have better-quality sleep, exercising at the same time every day will also help to set a regular pattern for your day.

- *Get out in the sun every afternoon,* even if it is only for fifteen or twenty minutes. The sun is necessary to keep your "body clock" correctly set.

- *Get used to doing the same things every night before going to bed.* This can be anything from watching the news, to reading a chapter of a book, to taking a warm bath. By developing and sticking to a getting-ready-for-bed routine, you will be telling your body that it's time to start winding down and relax.

But I can't fall (back) asleep

- *Use your bed and your bedroom only for sleeping and for sex.* If you get into bed and find that you can't fall asleep, get out of bed and go into another room until you begin to feel sleepy again.

- *Don't keep a TV set in the bedroom.* People often have a TV set in the bedroom, thinking that it helps them fall asleep. It doesn't. It actually keeps the mind racing and interferes with sleep. You might think, "But I always fall asleep with the TV on!" But do you ever fall asleep *early* with it on? Not likely. You probably fall asleep while the late show is on!

- *Refocus your mind away from worries.* You may get to sleep without a problem, but then wake up with the "early morning worries"—you can't turn off your mind. Then you get more worried because you cannot go back to sleep once you have awakened. Keeping your mind occupied with something else will ward off the worries and help you get back to sleep. For example, try quieting your mind by counting backward from 100 by threes or naming a flower for every letter of the alphabet.

- *Don't worry excessively about not getting enough sleep.* If your body needs sleep, you will sleep. Set yourself up for sleeping success but don't beat yourself up about missing an hour or two. Also, remember that people tend to need less sleep as they get older.

STRESS

Stress is a common problem for everyone. But what is stress? In the 1950s, physiologist Hans Selye described stress as "the nonspecific response of the body to any demand made upon it." Others have expanded this definition to define stress as the body's adaptation to demands, whether pleasant or unpleasant.

How Does Your Body Respond to Stress?

Your body is used to functioning at a certain level. When there is a need to change this level, your body must adjust physiologically to meet the demand. Your body reacts by preparing itself to take an action: Your heart rate increases, your blood pressure rises, your neck and shoulder muscles tense, your breathing becomes more rapid, your digestion slows, your mouth becomes dry, and you may begin sweating. These are typical signals of stress.

What causes stress responses?

To take an action, your muscles need a supply of oxygen and energy. Your rate of breathing increases in an effort to inhale as much oxygen as possible and to get rid of as much carbon dioxide as possible. Your heart rate increases to deliver the oxygen and nutrients to the muscles.

How long will the stress responses last?

In general, stress responses are present only until the stressful event passes. Your body then returns to its normal level of functioning. Sometimes, though, your body does not return to its former comfortable level. If the stress is present for any length of time, your body begins adapting to this stress. This adaptation can contribute to the development of health problems such as hypertension (high blood pressure) and shortness of breath.

Common Types of Stressors

Regardless of the type of stressor (a stressor is the thing that causes a stress response), the changes in the body are the same. Stressors, however, are not completely independent of one another. In fact, one stressor can often lead to other types of stressors or even magnify existing stressors. Several stressors can also occur at the same time. This works in much the same way as the vicious cycle of deconditioning and helplessness, described in Chapter 1.

These are some of the more common sources and types of stress:

- *Physical stressors.* Physical stressors can range from something as pleasant as going out dancing, or as common as grocery shopping, to something unpleasant, like the physical symptoms of your HIV/AIDS. The one thing that these three stressors have in common is that they all increase your body's demand for energy. If your body is not prepared to deal with this demand, the results may be sore muscles, fatigue, and a worsening of some disease symptoms.

- *Mental and emotional stressors.* Mental and emotional stressors can range from pleasant to uncomfortable. The joys you experience in seeing your sister get married or meeting new friends induce the same stress response in the body as feeling frustrated or "down" because of your illness. Although it seems strange that this is true, the difference comes in the way the stress is perceived by your brain.

- *Environmental stressors.* Environmental stressors can also be good or bad. They may be as varied as a sunny day, uneven sidewalks that make it difficult to walk, loud noises, or secondhand smoke.

Recognizing When You Feel Stressed

In reality, you have a certain need for stress—it helps your life run more efficiently. As long as you don't go past your breaking point, stress is helpful. On some days you can tolerate more stress than on others. But sometimes, if you are not aware of the different types of stress you are experiencing, you can go beyond your breaking point and feel like your life is completely out of control. It is often difficult to recognize when you are under too much stress.

The warning signs of stress include:

- Biting your nails, pulling your hair, or other repetitive habits

- Grinding your teeth, clenching your jaw

- Tension in your head, neck, or shoulders (which can cause headaches)

- Feelings of anxiousness, nervousness, helplessness, or irritability

Sometimes you can catch yourself engaging in these stress responses. If you do, take a few minutes to think about what it is that is making you feel tense. Take a few deep breaths and try to relax. Some methods for using your mind to help you relax are presented in Chapter 10, "Using Your Mind to Manage Symptoms."

Dealing with Stress

Stress can't be "cured," because it's part and parcel of everyday life. But you can learn to deal with the bad effects of stress. Two ways of coping with stress are: (1) avoiding stressful situations; and (2) managing stressful situations.

Avoiding stressful situations

Some situations are immediately identifiable as stressful; for example, being stuck in traffic, going on a trip, preparing meals, or going to a job interview. First, look—as objectively as possible—at what it is about the particular situation that is stressful. Is it that you hate to be late? Are trips stressful because of the uncertainty involved with your destination? Does meal preparation involve too many steps that demand too much energy?

Once you have determined what specifically is stressful about a situation, you can begin looking for ways to avoid the aspects of the situation that are creating stress for you. Can you leave earlier? Can you let someone else drive? Can you call someone at your destination site and ask about wheelchair access, local mass transit, and so on? Can you prepare food in the morning? Can you take a short nap in the early afternoon? After you have identified some possible solutions, select one to try the next time you are in this situation. Don't forget to evaluate the results. (This is the problem -solving approach we discuss in Chapter 2, "Becoming an HIV/AIDS Self-Manager.")

Managing the stress

Although you can successfully manage some types of stress by avoiding the stressful parts of the situation, many other types of stress seem to sneak up on you when you don't expect them. Dealing with this type of stress also involves the problem-solving approach.

If you know that certain situations will be stressful, develop ways to deal with them before they happen. Try to rehearse in your mind what you will do when the situation arises. Inherent in this approach is listening to your body for signals that the tension and stress are building. The better you become at listening to and understanding your body's signals, the better you'll become at managing your stress and stressful situations.

Certain chemicals, such as nicotine, alcohol, and caffeine, can also increase stress. Although you may smoke a cigarette, drink a glass of wine, or drink a cup of coffee to soothe your tension, these substances, in fact, actually increase the stress response in your body. Eliminating these stressors can leave you feeling calmer.

Chapter 10, "Using Your Mind to Manage Symptoms," discusses mental techniques, such as self-talk, progressive muscle relaxation, guided imagery, and visualization, which may also be useful to you in stressful situations. Other ways to deal with stress, such as getting enough sleep, exercising, and eating well, are discussed in this chapter and in Chapters 11 and 12.

In summary, stress, like every other symptom, has many causes and, therefore, has more than one way to be managed. It is up to you to examine the problem and try those solutions that meet your needs and lifestyle.

Taking actions to physically deal with your symptoms is necessary in coping with your illness on a day-to-day basis. But sometimes this just doesn't seem to be enough. There are times during the day when you may wish to escape from your surroundings and just have "your time"—a time that allows you to clear your mind, to gain a fresh perspective. The following chapter will show you different ways to complement your physical symptom management with cognitive techniques—techniques in which you use your mind to help reduce and even prevent some of the symptoms commonly experienced with HIV/AIDS.

SUGGESTED READING

Ball, Nigel, and Hough, Nick. *The Sleep Solution: A 21-Night Program for Restful Sleep.* Berkeley, Calif.: Ulysses Press, 1998.

Faelten, Sharon, and Diamond, David. *Tension Turnaround: 30-Day Program for Inner Calm, Confidence and Control.* Emmaus, Penn.: Rodale Press, 1990.

Kleinke, Chris L. *Coping with Life Challenges.* 2nd ed. Long Grove, Ill.: Waveland Press, 2002.

Natelson, Benjamin H. *Facing and Fighting Fatigue: A Practical Approach.* New Haven, Conn.: Yale University Press, 1998.

Zammit, Gary, and Zanca, Jane A. *Good Nights: How to Stop Sleep Deprivation, Overcome Insomnia and Get the Sleep You Need.* Kansas City, Mo.: Andrews & McMeel, 1998.

CHAPTER TEN

Using Your Mind to Manage Symptoms

All of us, at one time or another, have experienced the power of the mind and its effects on the body. Our thoughts and feelings, both pleasant and unpleasant, can cause the body to react in different ways. Often the heart rate and breathing are affected. We may also experience other sensations such as perspiration, warm or cold, blushing, or tears. Sometimes just a memory or image can create these responses. For example, take a moment now and think about a big, juicy lemon. Now think about sucking on the lemon. What happens? Your mouth puckers and starts to water. You may even smell the scent of the lemon. All of these reactions are triggered by the mind and its memory of a lemon.

This example demonstrates the power of the mind over the body and why it pays to develop our mental abilities to help us manage the different symptoms of HIV/AIDS. Through training and practice, we can learn to use the mind to relax the body, reduce stress, and decrease the discomfort caused by physical and emotional symptoms. The mind can also help to relieve pain and shortness of breath, and may even help you depend less on medications to relieve your symptoms.

In this chapter we describe several ways, called cognitive techniques, in which you can use your mind to manage symptoms.

RELAXATION TECHNIQUES

Although you may have heard and read about relaxation, you may still be confused as to what it is, what its benefits are, and how to do it. Relaxation is not a cure-all, but can be an effective part of treatment. There are different types of relaxation techniques, each with specific guidelines and uses. Some techniques are used only to achieve muscle relaxation; others are aimed at reducing anxiety and emotional arousal, or at diverting attention, all of which aid in symptom management.

The term *relaxation* means different things to different people. We can all identify ways we relax. For example, we may walk, watch TV, listen to music, cook, or garden. These methods of relaxing, however, are different from the techniques discussed here because they include some form of physical activity that requires your mind's attention. Relaxation techniques are also different from taking a nap or resting because we are using the mind actively to help the body achieve a relaxed state. The goal of relaxation is to turn off the outside world so the mind and body are at rest. This state allows you to reduce the tension that can increase the intensity of symptoms. When you have become adept at using the relaxation techniques described here, you will find that your relaxation sessions leave you with an overall feeling of peace and well-being, and a lessening of your physical symptoms.

MUSCLE RELAXATION

Muscle relaxation is one of the most commonly used cognitive techniques for symptom management. It is popular because it makes sense to us. If we are told that physical stress or muscular tension intensifies our pain, shortness of breath, or emotional distress, we are motivated to learn how to recognize this tension and release it. In addition, muscle relaxation is easy to learn and practice in different situations. It is one technique in which we can recognize some immediate results, such as the positive sensations of reduced pain, stress, or muscle tension, and calm, normal breathing. Muscle relaxation is not likely to fail because of distractions caused by symptoms or thoughts. It is a useful strategy to reduce pain, muscular tension, and stress while helping to control shortness of breath and achieve a more restful sleep.

Here we describe two muscle relaxation techniques. Try both techniques and choose the one that works best for you. Then tape-record the script for that routine. Although recording the script is not necessary, it may be helpful if you find it hard to concentrate. Also, you won't be distracted by having to refer to the book when you are trying to relax.

GUIDELINES FOR RELAXATION TECHNIQUES

- *Pick a quiet place and time* during the day when you will not be disturbed for at least 15–20 minutes. (If this seems too long, start with 5 minutes.)

- *Try to practice the technique twice daily*, but not less than four times a week.

- *Don't expect miracles.* Some of these techniques require time to acquire the skill. Three to four weeks of consistent practice may be needed before you really notice benefits.

- *Relaxation should be helpful.* At worst, you may find it boring; but if it is an unpleasant experience or makes you more nervous or anxious, then you should try one of the other symptom-management techniques described in this chapter.

Progressive Muscle Relaxation

Many years ago, a physiologist named Edmund Jacobson discovered that in order to relax, one must know how it feels to be tense, as well as relaxed. He believed that if one learned to recognize tension, then one could learn to let it go and relax. He designed a simple exercise to assist with this learning process.

To relax muscles, you need to know how to scan your body, recognize where you are holding tension, and release that tension. The first step is to become familiar with the difference between the feeling of tension and the feeling of relaxation. The brief progressive muscle relaxation exercise on the following pages will allow you to compare those feelings and, with practice, identify and release tension anywhere in your body.

As Jacobson emphasizes in the exercise, the purpose of voluntarily tensing the muscles is to learn to recognize and locate tension in your body. You will then become aware of tension and be able to use this same procedure to let it go. Once you learn the technique, it will no longer be necessary to tense voluntarily—just locate the existing tension and let it go.

For some people with a lot of pain, particularly in the joints, the Jacobson progressive muscle relaxation technique may not be appropriate. If it causes any pain, the pain may distract you from the relaxation. If this is the case, the body scan technique may work better for you.

Body Scan

The body scan is a relaxation technique similar to Jacobson's progressive muscle relaxation exercise, but it doesn't require the tensing or movement of muscle groups. Like Jacobson's exercise, it is best done while lying on your back, but any comfortable position can be used. First, you must focus on your breathing. Spend a few minutes concentrating on each breath as it enters and leaves your body. Try directing your breath past your chest, all the way down to your abdomen. (This is diaphragmatic breathing, described in Chapter 9, "Understanding the Symptom Cycle," and is an important part of all relaxation exercises.)

After three or four minutes of concentrating on your breathing, put your attention on your toes. Don't move the toes; just think about how they feel. Don't worry if you don't feel anything at all. If you find any tension there, let it go as you breathe out.

After a few moments of concentrating on your toes, move your attention to the bottoms of your feet. Again, don't move; just concentrate on any sensations you may have. Let go of any tension as you breathe out. Next, concentrate on the tops of your feet and your ankles. After a few more moments, bring your attention to your lower legs.

Continue this process, shifting your attention every few moments to another part of your body, working slowly upward to your head. If you find tension, let it go as you breathe out. If your mind starts to wander, just bring your attention back to the feelings in your body and to your breathing.

This technique can also be used to help you get to sleep, because it helps to clear your mind of any worries or distracting thoughts. The key is to give your full attention to scanning your body for tension and releasing it.

IMAGERY AND VISUALIZATION TECHNIQUES

Although relaxation techniques are the most common methods used to reduce muscle tension and stress, other cognitive techniques can also be useful. Techniques such as imagery and visualization can help to reduce fear, worry, and anxiety and take your mind off the unpleasantness of your symptoms.

Guided Imagery

The guided imagery relaxation technique is like a guided daydream. It allows you to refocus your mind away from your symptoms by transporting you to another time and place. It has the added benefit of helping you to achieve deep relaxation by picturing yourself in a peaceful environment. The guided imagery script presented in the following pages can help take you on this mental stroll.

There are several ways in which you can use the guided imagery script:

- You can read the script over several times to become familiar with it. Then sit or lie down in a quiet place and try to reconstruct the scene in your mind. Each script should take ten to fifteen minutes to complete.

- You can have a family member or friend read you the script slowly, pausing for five to ten seconds wherever there is a series of dots (. . .).

- You can make a tape of the script and play it to yourself whenever it's convenient.

PROGRESSIVE MUSCLE RELAXATION EXERCISES

This exercise guides you through the major muscle groups, asking you to first tense and then relax those muscles. If you have pain in a particular area, tense those muscles only gently or not at all, and focus on relaxing them.

1. Make yourself as comfortable as possible. Loosen any clothing that feels tight. Uncross your legs and ankles. Allow your body to feel supported by the surface on which you are sitting or lying.

2. Close your eyes. Take a deep breath, filling your chest and breathing all the way down to the abdomen. Hold . . . . Breathe out through pursed lips, and as you breathe out, let as much tension as possible flow out with your breath. Let all your muscles feel heavy and let your whole body just sink into the surface beneath you . . . . Good.

3. Become aware of the muscles in your feet and calves. Pull your toes back up toward your knees. Notice the tension in your feet and calves. Release and relax. Notice the discomfort leaving as relief and warmth replace it. That's it.

4. Now tighten the muscles of your thighs and buttocks. Hold and feel the tension. Let go and allow the muscles to relax. The relaxed muscles feel heavy and supported by the surface upon which you are sitting or lying.

5. Tense the muscles in your abdomen and chest. Notice a tendency to hold your breath as you tense. Relax, and notice that it is natural to want to take a deep breath to relieve the tension in this area. Take a deep breath now, breathing all the way down to the abdomen. As you breathe out, allow all the tension to flow out with your breath.

CONTINUED ON NEXT PAGE

> ### PROGRESSIVE MUSCLE RELAXATION EXERCISES (CONTINUED)
>
> 6. Now, stretching your fingers out straight, tense your fingers and tighten your arm muscles. Relax. Feel the tension flowing out as the circulation returns.
>
> 7. Press your shoulder blades together, tightening the muscles in your shoulders and neck. This is an area where many people carry a lot of tension. Hold . . . . Now, let go. Notice how the muscles feel warmer and more alive.
>
> 8. Tighten all the muscles of your face and head. Notice the tension, especially around your eyes and in your jaw. Now relax, allowing your jaw to become slack and your mouth to remain slightly open . . . . That's right. Note the difference.
>
> 9. Now take another deep breath, breathing all the way down to the abdomen. And, as you breathe out, allow your body to sink heavily into the surface beneath you, becoming even more deeply relaxed. Good.
>
> 10. Enjoy this comfortable feeling of relaxation. . . . Remember it. With practice, you will become skilled at recognizing muscle tension and releasing it.
>
> 11. Prepare to come back to the here and now. Take three deep breaths. When you're ready, open your eyes.

Visualization

Visualization, also referred to as *vivid imagery*, is similar to guided imagery. It is another way of using your imagination to picture yourself any way you want, doing things you want to do. You can practice visualization in different ways and for longer, as well as brief, periods. You can also use this relaxation technique while you are engaged in other activities.

One way to use visualization is to recall pleasant scenes from your past or to create new scenes in your mind. It allows you to create more of your own images than the guided imagery technique does. For example, try to remember every detail of a special holiday or party that made you happy. Who was there? What happened? What did you talk about? You can do the same sort of thing by remembering a vacation. In fact, visualization can be used to plan the details of some future event or to fill in the details of a pleasant fantasy. For example, how would you spend a million dollars? What would be your ideal romantic encounter? What would your ideal home or garden look like? Where would you go and what would you do on your dream vacation?

Another form of visualization involves imagining symbols that represent the discomfort or pain you feel in different parts of your body. For example, a painful joint might be red, or a tight chest might have a constricting band around it. After forming these images, you then try to change them. The red color might fade until there is no more color, or the constricting band might stretch and stretch until it falls off. Visualization is also a useful technique to help you set and accomplish your personal goals. (See Chapter 2, "Becoming an HIV/AIDS Self-Manager.") After you write your weekly action plan, take a few minutes to imagine yourself taking a walk, doing your exercises, or taking your medications. Here you are mentally rehearsing the steps you need to take in order to carry out your action plan. Studies have shown that this technique can help people cope better with stressful situations, master skills, and accomplish personal goals. In fact, people who have become skilled at visualization find that they can actually decrease some of the discomfort and distress associated with symptoms by changing unpleasant images to pleasant ones.

All the relaxation techniques mentioned above can be used in conjunction with pursed-lip and diaphragmatic breathing. These breathing techniques, described in Chapter 9, "Understanding the Symptom Cycle," can help you achieve a more relaxed state and keep your mind off any potential for shortness of breath.

A WALK IN THE COUNTRY (GUIDED IMAGERY)

- Make yourself as comfortable as possible, sitting or lying down. Loosen any constricting clothing. Uncross your arms, legs, and ankles. Allow your body to feel supported by the surface on which you are sitting or lying.

- Close your eyes.

- Take a deep breath, in through your nose, breathing all the way down to the abdomen. Hold . . . . Breathe out slowly through slightly pursed lips. As you do, relax your whole body, allowing all your muscles to feel limp and heavy . . . . Good.

- Scan your body for any muscle tension, starting with your head and going all the way down to your toes.

- Release any tension in your face, head, and neck by letting your jaw become slack and your head feel heavy on your shoulders. Allow your shoulders to drop heavily. Take a deep breath and relax your chest and abdomen. Allow your arms and legs to feel heavy and to sink into the surface beneath you.

- Now take a deep breath and become aware of any remaining tension in your body. As you breathe out, allow all the muscles of your body to sink heavily into the surface beneath you, becoming even more deeply relaxed . . . . Good.

- Imagine yourself walking along an old country road . . . the sun is warm on your back . . . the birds are singing . . . the air is calm and fragrant.

- As you progress down the road, you come across an old gate . . . . The gate creaks as you open it and go through.

- You find yourself in an overgrown garden, flowers growing where they have seeded themselves, vines climbing over a fallen tree, green grass, shade trees.

CONTINUED ON NEXT PAGE

A WALK IN THE COUNTRY (GUIDED IMAGERY) (CONTINUED)

- Breathe deeply, smelling the flowers . . . listen to the birds and insects . . . feel the gentle breeze, warm against your skin.

- As you walk leisurely up a gentle slope behind the garden, you come to a wooded area where the trees become denser and the sun is filtered through the leaves. The air feels mild and a bit cooler. You become aware of the sound and fragrance of a nearby brook. You breathe deeply of the cool and fragrant air several times, and with each breath you feel more refreshed.

- Soon you come upon the brook. It is clear and clean as it tumbles over the rocks and some fallen logs. You follow the path along the brook for a ways. The path takes you out into a sunlit clearing where you discover a small, picturesque waterfall . . . . There is a rainbow in the mist . . . .

- You find a comfortable place to sit for a while, a perfect niche where you feel completely relaxed.

- You feel good as you allow yourself to just enjoy the warmth and solitude of this peaceful place.

- It is now time to return. You walk back down the path, through the cool and fragrant trees, out into the sun-drenched overgrown garden . . . . One last smell of the flowers, and out the creaky gate . . .

- You leave this secret retreat for now and return down the country road. However, you know that you may visit this special place whenever you wish.

- When you are ready, take three deep breaths and open your eyes whenever you wish.

OTHER COGNITIVE STRATEGIES

Other cognitive strategies, such as distraction, self-talk, meditation, and reflection, take a different approach to managing symptoms. These techniques all involve retraining your patterns of thinking so that symptoms seem less intense, less limiting, or less important.

Distraction

Because the mind has trouble focusing on more than one thing at a time, you can lessen the intensity of your symptoms by training your mind to focus on something other than your body and its sensations. This technique, called *distraction* or *attention refocusing,* is particularly helpful if you feel your symptoms are overwhelming or worry that every bodily sensation might indicate a new or worsening symptom or health problem. It is important to note that with distraction you are not ignoring the symptoms, but choosing not to dwell on them.

Distraction works best for short activities or episodes in which symptoms may be anticipated, as in the following examples:

- *Make plans for exactly what you will do after the unpleasantness passes.* For example, if you have trouble falling asleep, try making plans for some future event, being as detailed as possible.

- *Think of a person's name, a bird, a flower, or other object for every letter of the alphabet.* If you get stuck on one letter, go on to the next. (These are good distractions for physical discomfort as well as for sleep problems.)

- *Count backward* from 1000 or 100 by threes (for example, 100, 97, 94, . . .).

- *Try to remember the words to a favorite song or the events in an old story.*

There are, of course, numerous variations to these examples, all of which will help you to refocus attention away from your problem.

So far we have discussed short-term distraction strategies in which you refocus your mind internally, away from your symptoms to thoughts of something more pleasant. There is another kind of distraction, the distraction of action, that works well for long-term projects or for symptoms that tend to last longer, such as depression and some forms of chronic pain. In this type of distraction, the mind is focused not internally but rather externally, on some type of activity. If you are slightly depressed or have continuous unpleasant symptoms, find an activity that interests you, and you will find yourself distracted from the problem. This activity can be almost anything, such as gardening, cooking, reading, going to a movie, or even doing volunteer work. One of the marks of a successful self-manager is that he or she has a variety of interests and always seems to be doing something.

Self-Talk: "I Know I Can"

We talk to ourselves all the time. For example, when waking up in the morning we may think, "I really don't want to get out of bed. I'm tired and don't want to go to work today." Or at the end of an enjoyable evening we think, "That was fun. I should get out more often." These things we think or say to ourselves are called *self-talk*.

All of our self-talk is learned from others and becomes a part of us as we grow up. It comes in many forms, most of which are negative. Negative self-statements usually take the form of: "I just can't do . . . ," "If only I could . . . ," "I just don't have the energy to . . . ." This type of self-talk represents the doubts and fears we have about ourselves in general and about our abilities to deal with a disease and its symptoms in particular. Unfortunately, negative self-talk can have the effect of worsening symptoms such as pain, depression, and fatigue.

Because what we learn in life influences our beliefs, attitudes, feelings, and actions, what we say to ourselves plays a major role in determining our success or failure in becoming good self-managers. Learning to make self-talk work *for* you instead of *against* you, by changing those negative statements to positive ones, will help you manage your symptoms more effectively. This change, as with any habit, requires practice.

To change negative self-talk to positive:

1. *Listen carefully to what you say to or about yourself, both out loud and silently.* Then write down all the negative self-talk statements. Pay special attention to the things you say during times that are particularly difficult for you. For example, what do you say to yourself when getting up in the

morning with pain, while doing those exercises you don't really like, or at those times when you are feeling blue?

2. *Work on changing each negative statement you identified to a positive one, and write these down.* Positive statements should reflect the better you and your decision to be in control. For example, negative statements such as "I don't want to get up," "I'm too tired and I hurt," "I can't do the things I like anymore so why bother," or "I'm good for nothing" become positive messages, such as "I have the energy to get up and do the things I enjoy," "I know I can do anything I believe I can," "People like me and I feel good about myself" or "Other people need and depend on me. I'm worthwhile."

3. *Read and rehearse these positive statements, mentally or with another person.* It is this conscious repetition or memorization of positive self-talk that will help you replace those old, habitual negative statements.

4. *Practice these new statements in real situations.* This practice, along with time and patience, will help your new patterns of thinking become automatic.

Once established, positive self-talk can be one of the most powerful tools you can add to your self-management program, helping you to manage symptoms as well as to master the other skills discussed in this book.

Mindfulness Meditation

There are many types of meditation. In fact, meditation is a part of most religious or spiritual traditions. The purpose of meditation is to quiet the mind. It can also help to quiet the body. For this reason, meditation is often a useful technique for managing stress and other symptoms, such as pain, fatigue, and shortness of breath. Mindfulness meditation is one type of meditation that can be practiced by anyone. All you need to begin is a quiet place and five minutes or more. Start by sitting in a chair with your feet flat on the floor and your hands in your lap or on your knees. If you wish and are able, sit on the floor with crossed legs or in a more traditional yoga position. How you sit, however, does not matter.

The essence of mindfulness meditation is to concentrate fully on your breathing. It is best if you can do diaphragmatic or belly breathing, but you do not have to take deep breaths. It is important to keep your full attention on your breathing. Breathe in slowly, hold the breath for a moment, and then breathe out slowly. At all times concentrate on your breathing.

Although this seems fairly simple, you will find that your mind easily wanders. This is called "having a monkey mind." As soon as you notice that your mind is wandering, bring your attention back to your breathing. At first you may not be able to attend to your breathing for more than a minute or two. You will improve, however, with practice.

When you are doing this type of meditation, you may become very aware of your body. For example, your eye may itch or you may become uncomfortable in your sitting position. When this happens, first do nothing but pay attention to your breathing. In many cases you will find that the discomfort goes away. If it continues, scratch the itch or change your position. Pay full attention to what you are doing. With mindfulness meditation it is important to be fully aware of what you are doing at each moment!

Like all other self-management techniques, mindfulness meditation requires practice. You will not get results immediately, but if you practice for fifteen to thirty minutes a day, four or five days a week, you will find that meditation can be a great symptom management tool.

Prayer or Reflection

Over the years, many people with chronic health problems have told us that prayer or reflection has been helpful in managing both the physical and emotional symptoms of their disease. For some, these practices are forms of relaxation that help reduce tension and anxiety. For others, these activities of the mind may be a method of distraction by which they refocus their attention or separate themselves from their symptoms. Regardless of the rationale, prayer and reflection are important parts of many people's self-management programs and are one of the oldest of all symptom management techniques.

As we mentioned earlier in this book, symptoms, their causes, and the ways they interact to affect your daily life can become a vicious cycle. It is important to identify these symptoms and their causes in order to break the cycle and become a successful self-manager. We close the chapter with some key principles to remember in the accompanying box.

PRINCIPLES OF SYMPTOM SELF-MANAGEMENT

- *Symptoms have many causes.* Thus, there are many ways to manage most symptoms. Understanding the nature and varied causes of your symptoms and how these interact will help you to better manage your symptoms.

- *Not all management techniques will work for everyone.* It is up to you to experiment and find out what works best for you. Be flexible. This includes trying different techniques and monitoring the results to see which technique is most helpful for which symptom(s) and under what circumstances.

- *Give yourself several weeks to practice a new symptom management technique before you decide whether it is working for you.* Remember that learning a new skill and gaining control of the situation take time.

- *Don't give up*, even if you feel you are not accomplishing anything. As is the case with exercise and other acquired skills, using your mind to manage your illness requires both practice and time before you notice the benefits. Be patient and keep on trying!

- *Self-management techniques should not have negative effects.* If you become frightened, angry, or depressed when using any one of these techniques, do not continue to use it. Try another technique instead.

SUGGESTED READING

Craze, Richard. *Teach Yourself Relaxation. New Edition.* London: Hodder & Stoughton, 2003.

Davis, Martha, Eshelman, Elizabeth Robbins, and McKay, Matthew. *The Relaxation and Stress Reduction Workbook.* Revised ed. Oakland, Calif.: New Harbinger Publications, 2000.

McKay, Matthew, and Fanning, Patrick. *The Daily Relaxer.* Oakland, Calif.: New Harbinger Publications, 1997.

McKay, Matthew, Fanning, Patrick, Honeychurch, Carole, and Sutker, Catherine. *The Self-Esteem Companion: Simple Exercises to Help Challenge Your Inner Critic and Celebrate Your Personal Strengths.* Oakland, Calif.: New Harbinger Publications, 1999.

Regan, Catherine. *Time for Healing: Relaxation for Mind and Body* (audio cassette or CD). Boulder, Colo.: Bull Publishing, 1994.

Rolek, Michiko J. *Mental Fitness: Complete Workouts for Body, Mind and Soul.* New York: Weatherhill, 1996.

PART FOUR

Managing Exercise and Diet

CHAPTER ELEVEN

Exercising for Fun and Fitness

Regular exercise and physical activity are vital to your physical and emotional health. They can also bring you fun and fitness. Having HIV/AIDS, however, can make it difficult to enjoy an active lifestyle. Some people may never have been really active, whereas others may have given up activities because of their condition or type of treatment. When you want to exercise but aren't sure what to do, physical and emotional limitations from HIV/AIDS can be powerful forces to overcome. Some people may even have been advised to avoid strenuous activity. Today, thanks to the knowledge gained from people with HIV/AIDS who have worked with health professionals in exercise research, we know it is safe to advise exercise for fun and fitness.

Traditional medical care of chronic illness has been based mainly on helping people when their illness worsened, and has involved recommendations to decrease physical activity and increase medical therapy. Unfortunately, long periods of inactivity in anyone can lead to weakness, stiffness, fatigue, poor appetite, constipation, high blood pressure, muscle loss, osteoporosis, and increased sensitivity to pain, anxiety, and depression. These inactivity-related problems can be caused by the illness itself or by medications, so it can be difficult to tell whether it is the illness, medication, inactivity, or a combination of the three that is responsible for these problems. Although we cannot cure HIV/AIDS yet, we do know that exercise can cure inactivity and have a positive effect on a number of HIV/AIDS-related problems. In this chapter we discuss the benefits of exercise and give you some pointers to get yourself started on self-managing your own fitness regime.

THE BENEFITS OF REGULAR EXERCISE

Exercise can help you maintain a healthy weight and improve your body composition, improve your appetite, and manage your blood sugar, fats, cholesterol, and blood pressure levels. Research has shown that people with HIV-related fatty deposits (lipodystrophy) can reduce fat by exercising. (See "A Note About Lipodystrophy," page 181.) In addition, exercise nourishes and strengthens your muscles and bones, helping to increase endurance and reduce fatigue. Regular exercise is also an important part of reducing the risks of complications for people who develop diabetes and high cholesterol from taking HAART medications. HIV/AIDS exercise studies have successfully used both endurance and strengthening exercise programs, frequently combining them for a complete fitness program.

Exercise is safe for people with HIV, and can have positive effects on the immune system, endurance, strength, and body fat. Short-term exercise has been shown to increase the numbers of T cells and other immune system cells in some HIV-positive people. In general people who are physically fit get fewer infections such as colds, and miss fewer days of work due to illness. Better fitness can lead to better mood, coping, and quality of life. Exercise conditions your body, helping to maintain cardiovascular and musculoskeletal fitness or restore function previously lost to disuse and illness. It will help you improve your health, feel better, and manage your illness better. Feeling more in control and less at the mercy of your illness is one of the biggest benefits of exercising.

If your illness is in a more active stage of HIV/AIDS, it is important to consult with your doctor and modify your exercise program as needed. Symptoms such as dizziness, vomiting, diarrhea, newly swollen joints, bleeding, or pain are reasons to cancel a workout until you can speak with your doctor. (See "Advice for Exercise Problems," page 215.)

This advice is not intended to take the place of specific therapeutic recommendations from your doctor or physical therapist. If an exercise plan has been prescribed for you that differs from the suggestions here, take this book to your doctor or physical therapist and ask what he or she thinks about this program.

DEVELOPING AN ACTIVE LIFESTYLE

One way to be more physically active is to set aside a time for a formal exercise program involving such planned activities as walking, jogging, swimming, tennis, dancing, or following an exercise videotape. These kinds of formal programs are what people usually think of when they think about exercise activity. But being more physical in everyday life can also pay off. Consider taking the stairs for a floor or two instead of waiting for the elevator. Park and walk the last few blocks to work or to the store instead of circling the parking lot looking for the perfect, up-close parking space. Play with the dog. Work in the garden. Just get up and walk around the house several times a day.

These types of daily activities, if done at moderate intensity and often enough, can result in significant health benefits. Recent studies show that even small amounts of daily activity can raise fitness levels in some people, and improve your health and mood—and the activities can be pleasurable, enjoyable ones! One person surveyed about activity level responded that she "*never* exercised." When asked about going dancing several times a week, she replied, "Oh, that's not exercise, that's fun." The average day is filled with excellent opportunities to be more physical and have more fun.

DEVELOPING AN EXERCISE PROGRAM

Although you can get lots of exercise from the activities of daily life, implementing a more formal exercise program can be helpful. Such a program usually involves setting aside a period of time, at least several times a week, to deliberately focus on increasing fitness.

A NOTE ABOUT LIPODYSTROPHY

Lipodystrophy is the movement of body fat from places you typically have had it, such as your buttocks, to places you may not have had it previously, such as your chest and stomach. (See Chapter 3, "Health Problems of People with HIV/AIDS," and Chapter 7, "Side Effects of Medications," for more on lipodystrophy-related health issues.) Although we do not understand the exact causes of lipodystropy, we believe it is associated with the following factors:

- Use of certain HIV drugs

- Age (it is more common in older people)

- Race (it is more common in Caucasians)

- Length of HIV infection (it is more common in people who have had HIV for a long time)

- Low T cell count

Besides changing the way your body looks and feels, lipodystrophy often goes hand in hand with high cholesterol and low insulin resistance. If this is the case for you, you will be more likely to have heart problems or diabetes. This means that it is important for you to discuss your concerns about lipodystrophy with your doctor.

Although we do not yet know how to prevent lipodystrophy, some studies suggest that exercise—especially strengthening exercise—may help to prevent or minimize it. The best current research indicates that weight training, which builds muscle, can help to change the ratio between muscle and fat, and thus combat the effects of lipodystrophy. You may want to go to a gym or health club whose staff are familiar with lipodystrophy. If you cannot find a fitness facility with trainers who know about this condition, follow the advice in this chapter, which is appropriate for all people with HIV/AIDS.

CONTINUED ON NEXT PAGE

A NOTE ABOUT LIPODYSTROPHY (CONTINUED)

First, a word of caution: Many health food stores, trainers, magazines, and even friends may try to get you to take supplements for lipodystrophy and other HIV-related conditions. Please resist, at least until you have done your own research. Many supplements contain steroids or other drugs that will not help and may even harm you. You may get the right drugs, but in the wrong dosage. It is important to talk with a knowledgeable health professional before trying supplements. Here are two excellent Web sites where you can find accurate, unbiased information:

www.projinf.org
(an American-based organization)

www.aidsmap.com
(a British-based organization)

A complete, balanced exercise program should help you improve these three aspects of fitness:

- *Flexibility.* This refers to the ability of the joints and muscles to move through a full, normal range of motion. Limited flexibility can cause pain, increase risk of injury, and make muscles less efficient. Flexibility tends to decrease with age and inactivity, but you can increase or maintain your flexibility by doing gentle flexibility or stretching exercises.

- *Strength.* Muscles need to be exercised to maintain their strength. With inactivity, they tend to weaken and shrink (atrophy). The weaker the muscles get, the less we feel like using them and the more inactive we tend to become, creating a vicious cycle. Some of the disability and lack of mobility in people with HIV/AIDS is caused by decreased muscle mass and weakness. Strengthening exercises can help maintain muscle, reduce body fat, and bring back strength and muscle health that has been lost.

- *Endurance.* Our ability to sustain activity depends on certain vital capacities. The heart and lungs must work efficiently to distribute oxygen-rich blood to the muscles. The muscles must be conditioned to extract and use the oxygen.

Aerobic (meaning "with oxygen") exercise conditions the heart, blood vessels, and muscles. This type of exercise uses the large muscles of your body in rhythmic, continuous activity. The most effective activities involve your whole body: walking, jogging, swimming, dancing, mowing the lawn, and so on. Aerobic exercise improves cardiovascular fitness, lessens the risk of heart attack, and helps control weight. Aerobic exercise also promotes a sense of well-being—easing depression and anxiety, promoting restful sleep, and improving mood and energy levels.

A GOOD FITNESS PROGRAM

A complete fitness program combines exercises to improve each of the three important aspects of fitness: flexibility, strength, and endurance. If you haven't exercised regularly in some time or have discomfort, stiffness, shortness of breath, or weakness that interferes with your daily activities, it is a good idea to talk with your health care providers before beginning your fitness program. Otherwise, start by choosing a number of flexibility and strengthening exercises that you are willing to do every day or every other day. Once you are able to exercise comfortably for at least ten minutes at a time, you are ready to add some endurance or aerobic activities.

Many people are uncertain about how to choose the right exercises and how to know what is best for them. The truth is that the best exercises are the ones that will help you do what you most want to do. Having a goal (something you want your exercise program to help you achieve) is the most important ingredient of a successful fitness program. Once you have a goal in mind, it is much easier to choose exercises that make sense for you.

If you don't see how exercise can be helpful to you personally, it will be hard to get excited about adding yet another task to your day. The steps below may help you get started.

Choose Your Goal and Make a Plan

1. *Choose as a goal something that you want to do* but don't or can't do now because of some physical problem. For example, you might want to take a hiking trip with friends, paint your house, or have enough energy to host a family celebration.

2. *Think about why you can't or don't enjoy doing it now.* Maybe it is because you get tired before everybody else or you are too weak or short of breath to complete the activity.

3. *Decide what you can do to overcome the problem.* For example, you can gradually increase your endurance by walking a comfortable distance two or three times a week. Or you might practice deep breathing and strengthening exercises for your arms to help you manage your shortness of breath and upper-body weakness.

4. *Design your exercise plan.* Choose no more than ten to twelve flexibility and strengthening exercises at first. Start by doing three to five repetitions of each, if you have not exercised for awhile. As you improve, increase the number of repetitions and the number of exercises you do. If you want to improve endurance, first choose an aerobic activity you like (such as walking, swimming, bicycling, or dancing). Start by doing this activity for short periods, or for whatever period you are comfortable with now, and build up gradually. Health and fitness take time to build, but every day that you exercise makes you healthier and brings you closer to being fit. That's why it is important to keep it up.

FLEXIBILITY EXERCISES

If you have not been exercising, if you have been ill and are recovering, or if some part of the body is giving you trouble, this is the time to start

TIPS FOR EXERCISING FOR FLEXIBILITY AND STRENGTH

- *Move slowly and gently.* Do not bounce or jerk. Such movements actually tighten and shorten muscles.

- To loosen tight muscles and limber up stiff joints, *stretch just until you feel tension*, hold for 5 to 10 seconds, and then relax.

- *Don't push your body until it hurts.* Stretching should feel good, not painful.

- *Start with no more than five repetitions of any exercise.* Take at least two weeks to increase to ten.

- Always do the *same number* of repetitions for your left side as for your right.

- *Breathe naturally.* Do not hold your breath. Count out loud to make sure you are breathing easily. (If you are holding your breath, you are probably trying too hard. Back off.)

- If you feel increased symptoms that last more than *two hours* after exercising, next time do fewer repetitions, or eliminate the exercise that seems to be causing the symptoms. *Don't quit exercising.*

- *All exercises should be adapted to individual needs.* If you are limited by muscle weakness or joint tightness, go ahead and do the exercise as completely as you can. The benefit of doing an exercise comes from moving toward a certain position, not from being able to complete the movement perfectly the first time. In some cases you may find that after awhile you can complete the movement. Other times you will continue to perform your own version.

on a flexibility exercise program. These exercises may seem simple, or not nearly at the level of challenge you were used to. But if you are not up to anything more strenuous at the moment, these are the right exercises for you, and will lead you safely to a more vigorous and varied exercise program.

The following exercises are organized from the head and neck down to the toes. Most of the upper-body exercises may be done either sitting or standing. Exercises done lying down can be performed on the floor or on a firm mattress. We have labeled the exercises that are particularly important for good posture "VIP" (*Very Important for Posture*).

You may enjoy creating a routine of exercises that flow together. Arrange them so you don't have to get up and down too often. Exercising to gentle, rhythmic music can also add to your enjoyment. (See "Tips for Exercising for Flexibility and Strength," page 184.)

Neck Exercises

1. Heads Up (VIP)

This exercise relieves jaw, neck, and upper back tension or pain, and improves posture. You can do it while driving, sitting at a desk, reading, or during an exercise session. Just sit or stand straight and gently slide your chin back. You'll feel the back of your neck lengthen and straighten. To help, put your finger on your nose and then draw straight back from your finger.

Clues for finding the correct position:

- Ear over shoulder, not out in front.

- Head balanced over neck and trunk, not in the lead.

- Back of neck vertical, not leaning forward.

- You may observe a bit of double chin.

2. Neck Stretch

In heads-up position (Exercise 1) and with your shoulders relaxed:

1. Turn slowly to look over your right shoulder. Then turn slowly to look over your left shoulder.

2. Tilt your head to the right and then to the left. Move your ear toward your shoulder. Do not move your shoulder up to your ear.

Don't do these exercises if they cause neck pain, or pain or numbness in your arms or hands.

Hand and Wrist Exercises

A good place to do hand exercises is at a table that supports your forearms. Do them after washing dishes, after bathing, or when taking a break from handwork. Your hands are warmer and more limber at these times.

3. Thumb Walk

Holding your wrist straight, form the letter "O" by lightly touching your thumb to each fingertip. After each "O," straighten and spread your fingers. Use the other hand to help if needed.

4. Good Morning Stretch

Start with hands in gentle fists, palms turned toward you, and wrists crossed. Breathe in and extend fingers while you uncross your arms and reach up as high as you can. Breathe out and relax.

5. Wand Exercise

If one or both of your shoulders are tight or weak, you may want to give yourself a "helping hand." This shoulder exercise and the Pat and Reach exercise that follows allow the arms to help each other.

Use a cane, yardstick, or mop handle as your "wand." Place one hand on each end and raise the wand as high overhead as possible. You might try this in front of the mirror. This exercise can be done standing, sitting, or lying down.

6. Pat and Reach

This double-duty exercise helps increase flexibility and strength for both shoulders. Raise one arm up over your head, and bend your elbow to pat yourself on the back. Move your other arm behind your back, bend your elbow, and reach up toward the other hand. Can your fingertips touch? Relax and switch arms. Can you touch on that side? For most people, one position will work better than the other.

Back and Abdominal Exercises

7. Knee-to-Chest Stretch

For a lower back stretch, lie on the floor with knees bent and feet flat. Bring one knee toward your chest, using your hands to help. Hold your knee near your chest for ten seconds and lower the leg slowly. Repeat with the other knee. You can also bring both knees to your chest at the same time if you wish. Relax and enjoy the stretch.

8. Pelvic Tilt (VIP)

This is an excellent exercise for the lower back. Lie on your back with knees bent, feet flat. Place your hands on your abdomen. Flatten the small of your back against the floor by tightening your stomach muscles and your buttocks. It helps to imagine bringing your pubic bone to your chin, or trying to pull your tummy in enough to zip a tight pair of trousers. Hold the tilt for five to ten seconds. Relax. Arch your back slightly. Relax and repeat the Pelvic Tilt. Keep breathing. Count the seconds out loud. Once you've mastered the Pelvic Tilt lying down, practice it sitting, standing, and walking.

9. Back Lift (VIP)

This exercise improves flexibility along your spine. Lie on your stomach and rise up onto your forearms. Keep your back relaxed, and keep your stomach and hips down. If this is comfortable, straighten your elbows. Breathe naturally and relax for at least ten seconds. If you have moderate to severe lower back pain, do not do this exercise unless it has been specifically prescribed for you.

10. Lower Back Rock and Roll

Lie on your back and pull your knees up to your chest with your hands behind the thighs. Rest in this position for ten seconds, then gently roll knees from one side to the other, rocking your hips back and forth. Keep your upper back and shoulders flat on the ground.

Hip and Leg Exercises

11. Hip Hooray

This exercise can be done standing or lying on your back. If you lie down, spread your legs as far apart as possible. Roll your legs and feet out like a duck, then in to be pigeon-toed, move your legs back together. If you are standing, move one leg out to your side as far as you can. Lead out with the heel and in with the toes. Hold onto a counter for support.

(Lying down)   (Standing)

12. Back Kick (VIP)

This exercise increases the mobility and strength of your hip. Hold onto a counter for support. Move the leg up and back, knee straight. Stand tall, and do not lean forward.

13. Ready-Go (VIP)

Stand with one leg slightly in front of the other. Have your heel on the floor, as if you were going to take a step with the front foot. Now tighten the muscles on the front of your thigh, making your knee firm and straight. Hold for a count of 10. Repeat with the other leg.

14. Hamstring Stretch

If you have unstable knees or a knee that curves backward when you stand up, do not do this exercise.

If you do have tight hamstrings, lie on your back, knees bent, feet flat. Grasp one leg at a time behind the thigh. Holding the leg out at arm's length, slowly straighten the knee. Hold the leg as straight as you can as you count to 10. You should feel a slight stretch at the back of your knee and thigh.

Be careful with this exercise. It's easy to overstretch and be sore.

15. Achilles Stretch

This exercise helps maintain flexibility in the Achilles tendon, the large tendon at the back of your ankle. Good flexibility helps reduce the risk of injury, calf discomfort, and heel pain. The Achilles Stretch is especially helpful for cooling down after walking or cycling, and for people who get cramps in the calf muscles.

Stand at a counter or against a wall. Place one foot in front of the other, toes pointing forward and heels on the ground. Lean forward, bend the knee of the forward leg, and keep the back knee straight, heel down. You will feel a good stretch in the calf. Hold the stretch for ten seconds. Do *not* bounce. Move gently.

If you have trouble with spasticity (muscle jerks) or standing balance, you can do a seated version of this exercise. Sit in a chair with feet flat on the floor. Keep your heels on the floor and slowly slide one foot back to bend your ankle and feel some tension in the back of your calf.

It's easy to get sore doing this exercise. If you've worn shoes with high heels for a long time, be particularly careful.

Ankle and Foot Exercises

Do these exercises sitting in a straight-backed chair with your feet bare. Have a bath towel and ten marbles next to you. These exercises are for flexibility, strength, and comfort. This is a good time to examine your feet and toes for signs of circulation or skin problems, and to check your nails to see if they need trimming.

16. Towel Grabber

Spread a towel out in front of your chair. Place your feet on the towel, with your heels near the edge closest to you. Keep your heels down and your feet slightly raised. Scoot the towel back underneath your feet by pulling it

with your toes. When you have scooted it as much as you can, reverse the toe motion and scoot the towel out again.

17. Marble Pick-Up

Do this exercise one foot at a time. Place several marbles on the floor between your feet. Keep your heel down, and pivot your toes toward the marbles. Pick up one marble with your toes and pivot your foot to drop the marble as far as possible from where you picked it up. Repeat until you have moved all the marbles. Reverse the process and return all the marbles to the starting position. If it's difficult to work with marbles, try other objects, such as jacks, dice, or wads of paper.

18. Foot Roll

Place a rolling pin (or a large dowel or closet rod) under the arch of your foot, and roll it back

and forth. It feels great and stretches the ligaments in the arch of the foot.

Whole-Body Exercises

19. The Stretcher

This exercise is a whole-body stretch to do lying on your back. Start the motion at your ankles as explained here, or reverse the process if you want to start with your arms first.

- Point your toes, and then pull your toes toward your nose. Relax.

- Bend your knees. Then flatten your knees and let them relax.

- Arch your back. Do the Pelvic Tilt (page 189). Relax.

- Breathe in and stretch your arms above your head. Breathe out and lower your arms. Relax.

- Stretch your right arm above your head, and stretch your left leg by pushing away with your heel. Hold for a count of 10. Switch to the other side and repeat.

Self-Tests for Flexibility

Whatever our goals, we all need to see that our efforts make a difference. Because an exercise program produces gradual change, it's often hard to tell whether the program is working and to recog- nize improvement. Choose several of these flexibility and strength tests to measure your progress. Not everyone will be able to do all the tests. Choose those that work best for you. Perform each test before you start your exercise program, and record the results. After every four weeks, do the tests again and check your improvement.

Arm Flexibility

Do Flexibility Exercise 6 (Pat and Reach) for both sides of the body. Ask someone to measure the distance between your fingertips.

Goal: Less distance between your fingertips.

Shoulder Flexibility

Stand facing a wall, with your toes touching the wall. One arm at a time, reach up the wall in front of you. Hold a pencil, or have someone mark how far you reached. Do this sideways, also, standing about three inches (8 cm) away from the wall.

Goal: To reach higher.

Hamstring Flexibility

Do Flexibility Exercise 14 (the Hamstring Stretch), one leg at a time. Keep your thigh perpendicular to your body. How much does your knee bend? How tight does the back of your leg feel?

Goal: Straighter knee and less tension in the back of the leg.

Ankle Flexibility

Sit in a chair with your bare feet flat on the floor and your knees bent at a 90° angle. Keep your heels on the floor. Raise your toes and the front of your foot. Ask someone to measure the distance between the ball of your foot and the floor.

Goal: One to two inches (3 to 5 cm) between your foot and the floor.

STRENGTHENING EXERCISES

Strengthening exercises make your muscles work against resistance and thus grow stronger. Once you can do flexibility exercises for fifteen minutes, you are ready to start a strength program.

Strengthening exercises should not be done more often than every other day. Your muscles use the day off to adapt to the exercise and grow stronger. We suggest that you start with three to five repetitions of each exercise (be sure to do the same number on *both* sides). You can add repetitions—or weight (*not both*)—every ten days to two weeks. Once you have reached ten to twelve repetitions, doing more repetitions will not be helpful. Add weight instead. Many people doing strengthening exercise use machines or dumb bells. This is fine—just go easy. (See "Tips for Exercising for Flexibility and Strength," page 184.) The following exercises will get you started and require little or no equipment.

1. Shoulder Blade Pinch (VIP)

This is a good exercise to strengthen the middle and upper back and to stretch the chest. Sit or stand with your head in heads-up position (page 185) and your shoulders relaxed. Raise your arms out to the sides with elbows bent. Pinch your shoulder blades together by moving your elbows as far back as you can. Hold briefly, then slowly move your arms forward to touch elbows. If this position is uncomfortable, lower your arms or rest your hands on your shoulders.

2. Back Lift (VIP)

To strengthen back muscles, lie on your stomach with your arms at your sides or overhead. Lift your head, shoulders, and arms. Do not look up. Keep looking down with your chin tucked in. Count out loud as you hold for a count of 10. Relax. You can also lift your legs, instead of your head and shoulders, off the floor. Lifting both ends of your body at once is fairly strenuous exercise. It may not be helpful for a person with back pain. (See illustration, page 190.)

3. Curl-Up

A Curl-Up is a good way to strengthen abdominal muscles. Lie on your back, knees bent, feet flat. Do the Pelvic Tilt (page 189). Slowly curl up to raise your head and shoulders. Uncurl back down, or hold for ten seconds and slowly uncurl. Breathe out as you curl up, and breathe in as you go back down. Do *not* hold your breath. If you have neck problems, or if your neck hurts when you do this exercise, try the Roll-Out (described below) instead. *Never* tuck your feet under a chair or have anyone hold your feet!

4. Roll-Out

This is another good abdominal strengthener, and is easy on the neck. Use it instead of the Curl-Up, or—if neck pain is not a problem—do them both.

- Lie on your back with knees bent and feet flat. Do the Pelvic Tilt (page 189), and hold your lower back firmly against the floor.

- Slowly and carefully, move one leg away from your chest as you straighten your knee. Move your leg out until you feel your lower back start to arch. When this happens, tuck your knee back to your chest. Reset your pelvic tilt and roll your leg out again. Breathe out as your leg rolls out. Do not hold your breath. Repeat with the other leg.

You are strengthening your abdominal muscles by holding your pelvic tilt against the weight of your leg. As you get stronger, you'll be able to straighten your legs farther and move both legs together.

5. Straight Leg Raises

This exercise strengthens the muscles that bend the hip and straighten the knee. Lie on your back, knees bent, feet flat. Straighten one leg. Tighten the muscle on top of that thigh, and straighten the knee as much as possible. Keeping the knee straight, raise your leg one to two feet (about 50 cm) off the floor. Do not arch your back. Hold your leg up and count out loud for ten seconds. Relax. Repeat with the other leg.

6. Knee Strengthener (VIP)

Strong knees are important for walking and standing comfortably. Sitting in a chair, straighten the knee by tightening the muscle on top of your thigh. Place your hand on your thigh and feel the muscle work. If you wish, make circles with your toes. As your knee strengthens, see if you can build up to holding your leg out for thirty seconds. Count out loud. Do *not* hold your breath.

7. Power Knees

This exercise strengthens the muscles that bend and straighten your knee. Sit in a chair and cross your legs at the ankles. Your legs can be almost straight, or you can bend your knees as much as you like. Try several positions. Push forward with your back leg, and press backward with your front leg. Exert pressure evenly so that your legs do not move. Hold and count out loud for ten seconds. Relax. Switch legs. Be sure to keep breathing. Repeat.

8. Tiptoes

This exercise will help strengthen your calf muscles and make walking, climbing stairs, and standing less tiring. It may also improve your balance. Hold on to a counter or table for support and go up onto your tiptoes. Hold for ten seconds. Slowly lower your feet back to the floor. How high you go is not as important as keeping your balance and controlling your ankles. It is easier to do both legs at the same time. If your feet are too sore to do the exercise from a standing position, start by doing it while sitting down. If this exercise makes your ankle jerk, leave it out of your exercise program. Talk to your therapist about other ways to strengthen the calf muscles.

ENDURANCE EXERCISE: HOW MUCH IS ENOUGH?

One of the biggest problems with endurance (aerobic) exercise is that it is easy to overdo, even for people who don't have HIV/AIDS. Inexperienced and misinformed exercisers think they have to work very hard for exercise to do any good. Exhaustion, sore muscles, painful joints, and shortness of breath are the consequences of jumping in too hard and too fast. As a result, some people may put aside their exercise programs indefinitely, thinking that exercise is just not meant for them.

There is no magic formula for determining how much exercise you need. *The most important thing to remember is that some is better than none. Even a few minutes of exercise several times per week can be very beneficial.* If you start slowly and increase your efforts gradually, it is likely that you will maintain your exercise program as a lifelong habit. Generally, it is better to begin your conditioning program by *under*doing rather than *over*doing.

Several studies suggest that the upper limit of benefit is about 200 minutes of moderate-intensity aerobic exercise per week. Doing more than that doesn't gain you much (and it increases your risk of injury). On the other hand, doing 100 minutes of exercise per week gets you about ninety percent of the benefit, whereas sixty minutes of aerobic exercise per week yields about seventy-five percent of the benefit. Sixty minutes is just fifteen minutes of mild aerobic exercise, four times a week!

Following are some general guidelines for the frequency, duration, and intensity of aerobic exercise.

- *Frequency.* Try to exercise three or four times a week. Taking every other day off gives your body a chance to rest and recover. We recommend that you rest at least one day per week.

- *Duration.* Keep in mind that you may not be able to exercise as long as you once could. Start with just a few minutes, and then gradually increase the duration of your aerobic activity to about thirty minutes a session. You can safely increase the time by alternating intervals of brisk exercise with intervals of rest or easy exercise. For example, after three to five minutes of brisk walking, do one to two minutes of easy strolling and then another three to five minutes of brisk walking. Then gradual-ly eliminate rest intervals until you can maintain twenty to thirty min-utes of brisk exercise. If thirty minutes seems too long, consider two sessions of ten to fifteen minutes each. Both approaches appear to improve fitness levels significantly.

- *Intensity.* Safe and effective endurance exercise should be done at no greater than moderate intensity. High-intensity exercise increases the risk of injury and causes discomfort, so not many people stick with it. Exercise intensity is measured by how hard you work. For a trained runner, completing a mile in twelve minutes is probably low-intensity exercise. For a person who hasn't exercised in a long time, a brisk ten-minute walk may be of moderate to high intensity. For person with severe physical limitations, one minute may be of moderate intensity.

Fatigue, lack of cardiovascular conditioning, and poor endurance are common challenges for people with HIV/AIDS. People who have had HIV/AIDS for quite a while also may be at more risk for cardiovascular and lung problems and anemia. These conditions can limit the amount of exercise that can be performed, but for most people, low- or moderate-intensity aerobic exercise is comfortable and safe.

Remember, these are just rough guidelines on frequency, duration, and intensity—not a rigid prescription. Listen to your own body. Sometimes you need to tell yourself (and maybe others) that enough is enough. More exercise is not necessarily better, especially if it gives you pain or discomfort.

Intensity Guidelines

You can determine your own individual intensity guidelines through sever-al intensity-monitoring techniques: the talk test, perceived exertion test, and monitoring your heart rate.

Talk Test

Talk to another person or to yourself, sing, or recite poems out loud while you exercise. Moderate-intensity exercise allows you to speak com-fortably. If you can't carry on a conversation or sing because you are breathing too hard or are short of breath, you're working too hard. Slow down. The talk test is an easy way to regulate exercise intensity.

If you have breathing problems, the talk test may not work for you. If this is the case, use the perceived exertion test.

Perceived Exertion Test

Another way to monitor intensity is to rate how hard you're working on a scale of 0 to 10. Zero, at the low end of the scale, is lying down, doing no work at all. Ten is equivalent to working as hard as possible—very hard work that you couldn't continue doing longer than a few seconds. Of course, you never want to exercise that hard! A good level for your aerobic exercise routine is between 3 and 6 on this scale. At this level, you'll usually perspire and breathe faster and more deeply than usual, and your heart will beat faster than normal, but you shouldn't feel pain.

Heart Rate

Monitoring your heart rate while exercising is another way to measure exercise intensity. The faster the heart beats, the harder you're working. (Your heart also beats fast when you are frightened or nervous, but here we're talking about how your heart responds to physical activity.) Endurance exercise at moderate intensity raises your heart rate into a range of between sixty and eighty percent of your safe maximum heart rate. The safe maximum heart rate declines with age, so your safe exercise heart rate gets lower as you get older. You can follow the general guidelines of the following Exercise Heart Rate chart, or you can calculate your individual exercise heart rate. Either way, you need to know how to take your pulse.

Take your pulse by placing the tips of your middle three fingers at your wrist below the base of your thumb. Feel around in that spot until you feel the pulsations of blood pumping with each heartbeat. Count how many beats you feel in fifteen seconds. Multiply this number by 4 to find out how fast your heart is beating in one minute. Start by taking your pulse whenever you think of it, and you'll soon learn the difference between your resting and exercise heart rates.

Exercise Heart Rate

Calculate your own ideal exercise heart rate by following these steps:

1. Subtract your age from 220:

   Example: *220 − 40 = 180*   *You*: 220 − _____ = _____

2. To find the *lower* end of your exercise heart rate range, multiply your answer in step 1 by 0.6.

   Example: *180 × 0.6 = 108*   *You*: _____ × 0.6 = _____

3 To find the *upper* end of your exercise heart rate range, *which you should not exceed*, multiply your answer in step 1 by 0.8.

   Example: *180 × 0.8 = 144*   *You*: _____ × 0.8 = _____

The exercise heart rate range in our example is from 108 to 144 beats per minute. What is yours?

Most people count their pulse for fifteen seconds, not a whole minute. To find your fifteen-second pulse, divide both numbers by 4. The person in our example should be able to count between twenty-seven and thirty-six beats in fifteen seconds while exercising.

EXERCISE HEART RATE	
Age Range	Exercise Pulse (Beats per 15 Seconds)
20–30	29–39
30–40	28–37
40–50	26–35
50–60	25–33
60–70	23–31
70–80	22–29
80+	16–24

The most important reason to know your ideal exercise heart rate range is so that you can learn to not exercise too vigorously. After you've done your warm-up and five minutes of endurance exercise, take your pulse. *If it's higher than the upper rate, don't panic.* Slow down a bit. Don't work so hard.

At first, some people have trouble keeping their heart rate within the ideal exercise heart rate range. Don't worry about that. Keep exercising at the level at which you're most comfortable. As you get more experienced and stronger, you will gradually be able to do more vigorous exercise while keeping your heart rate within your "goal" range. But don't let the target heart rate monitoring become a burden. Recent studies have shown that even low-intensity exercise can provide significant health benefits. So use the ideal heart rate range as a rough guide, and don't worry if you can't reach the lower end of that range. The important thing is to keep exercising!

If you are taking medicine that regulates your heart rate, have trouble feeling your pulse, or think that keeping track of your heart rate is a bother, use one of the other methods to monitor your exercise intensity.

Self-Tests for Endurance and Aerobic Fitness

For some people, just the feelings of increased endurance and well-being are enough to indicate progress. Others may find it helpful to demonstrate that their exercise program is making a measurable difference. You may wish to try one or both of the following endurance and aerobic fitness tests before you start your exercise program. Not everyone will be able to do both tests, so pick the one that works best for you. Record your results in your exercise diary. After four weeks of exercise, do the test again and check your improvement. Measure your progress again after four more weeks.

When to Warm Up and Cool Down

If you are going to exercise at an intensity that causes you to breathe harder or your heart to beat faster, it is important to warm up first. A warm-up means that you do at least five minutes of a low-intensity activity to allow your heart, lungs, and circulation to gradually increase their work. If you are going for a brisk walk, first warm up with five minutes of slow walking.

DISTANCE SELF-TEST

- Find a place to walk or bicycle where you can measure distance. A running track works well. On a street, you can measure distance with a car. A stationary bicycle with an odometer provides the equivalent measurement. If you plan on swimming, you can count pool lengths.

- After a warm-up, note your starting point and either bicycle, swim, or walk as briskly as you comfortably can for five minutes. Try to move at a steady pace for the full time. At the end of five minutes, mark your spot and immediately take your pulse and rate your perceived exertion from 0 to 10. Continue at a slow pace for three to five more minutes to cool down. Measure and record the distance, your heart rate, and your perceived exertion.

- Repeat the test after several weeks of exercise. There may be a change in as little as four weeks. However, it often takes eight to twelve weeks to see improvement.

Goal: To cover more distance, lower your heart rate, or lower your perceived exertion.

If you are riding a stationary bike, warm up with five minutes of no resistance at no more than 60 rpm. In an aerobic exercise class, you will warm up with a gentle routine before moving on to more vigorous activity. Warming up reduces the risk of injury, soreness, and irregular heartbeat.

A cool-down period is important after you have exercised at an intensity that has made you breathe harder, feel warm or perspire, or caused your heart to beat faster. Repeating the five-minute warm-up activity or taking a slow walk helps your muscles to relax gradually, and your heart and breathing to slow down. Gentle flexibility and strengthening exercises during the cool-down can help increase your range of motion and reduce muscle soreness and stiffness.

TIME SELF-TEST

- Measure a given distance to walk, bike, or swim. Estimate how far you think you can go in one to five minutes. You can pick a number of blocks, actual distance, or lengths in a pool.

- Spend three to five minutes warming up. Start timing and start moving steadily, briskly, and comfortably. At the finish, record how long it took you to cover your course, your heart rate, and your perceived exertion.

- Repeat after several weeks of exercise. You may see changes in as little as four weeks. However, it often takes eight to twelve weeks for a noticeable improvement.

Goal: To complete the course in less time, at a lower heart rate, or at lower perceived exertion.

You may enjoy a routine of flexibility and strengthening exercises that you can use as part of your warm-up and cool-down periods. If you do, arrange the exercises so that they flow together and you don't have to get up and down too much. Also, try exercising to gentle, rhythmic music to make it more enjoyable.

WHAT ARE YOUR EXERCISE BARRIERS?

Fitness makes sense. Yet, when faced with the prospect of actually becoming more physically active, most people can come up with scores of excuses, concerns, and worries. These barriers can prevent us from even taking the first step. Following are some common barriers and possible solutions.

I don't have enough time.

Everyone has the same amount of time; we just choose to use it differently. It's a matter of priorities. Some find a lot of time for television, but none to spare for fitness. It doesn't really take a lot of time to become more active. Even five minutes a day is a good start, and much better than no physical activity. You may be able to combine activities, such as watching television while pedaling a stationary bicycle, or arranging "walking meetings" to discuss business or family matters.

I'm too tired.

When you're out of shape, you feel listless and tend to tire easily. Then you don't exercise because you're tired, and this becomes a vicious cycle. You have to break out of the too-tired cycle. Regular physical activity increases your stamina and gives you more energy to do the things you like. As you get back into shape, you will recognize the difference between feeling listless or out of shape and feeling physically tired.

I'm too sick.

It may be true that you are too sick for a vigorous or strenuous exercise program, but you can still usually find some ways to be more active. Remember, you can exercise one minute at a time, several times a day. The enhanced physical fitness you will gain can help you better cope with your illness and prevent further problems.

I get enough exercise.

This may be true, but for most people, their jobs and daily activities do not provide enough sustained exercise to keep them fully fit and energetic. Do you get at least one hundred minutes of endurance exercise each week?

Exercise is boring.

You can make it more interesting and fun. Exercise with other people. Entertain yourself with headphones and music, or listen to the radio. Vary your activities and your walking routes.

Exercise is painful.

The old saying, "No pain, no gain," is simply wrong and out of date. Recent evidence shows that significant health benefits come from gentle, low-intensity, enjoyable physical activity. You may sweat or feel a bit short of breath, but if you feel more pain than before you started, something is probably wrong. More than likely you are either exercising improperly or you're overdoing it. Talk with your physician. You may simply need to be less vigorous or change the type of exercise that you're doing.

I'm too embarrassed.

For some, the thought of donning a skin-tight designer exercise outfit and trotting around in public is delightful, but for others it is downright distressing. Fortunately, the options for physical activity range from exercise in the privacy of your own home to group social activities. You should be able to find something that suits you.

It's too cold, it's too hot, it's too dark . . .

If you are flexible and vary your type of exercise, you can generally work around the changes in weather that make certain types of exercise more difficult. Consider indoor activities such as stationary bicycling, exercising with a workout tape or DVD at home, or working out at the gym.

I'm afraid I won't be able to do it right or be successful. I'm afraid I'll fail.

Many people don't want to start a new project because they are afraid they will fail or not be able to finish it successfully. If you feel this way about starting an exercise program, remember two things. First, whatever activities you are able to do—no matter how short or "easy"—will be much better for you than doing nothing. Be proud of what you have done, not guilty about what you haven't done. Second, new projects often seem overwhelming—until you get started and learn to enjoy each day's adventures and successes. (See "Implementing a Successful Fitness Program," page 213.)

Perhaps you have come up with some other barriers. The human mind is incredibly creative. You can turn that creativity to your advantage by using it to come up with even better ways to refute the excuses, and to develop positive attitudes about exercise and fitness. If you get stuck, ask others for suggestions, or try some of the self-talk suggestions in Chapter 10, "Using Your Mind to Manage Symptoms."

OPPORTUNITIES IN YOUR COMMUNITY

Most people who exercise regularly do so with at least one other person. Two or more people can keep each other motivated, and a whole class can build a feeling of camaraderie. On the other hand, exercising alone gives you the most freedom. You may feel that there are no classes that would work for you, or no buddy with whom you can exercise. If so, start your own program; as you progress, you may find that these feelings change and you may eventually want to include others in your exercise plans.

Many communities now offer a variety of exercise classes, including special programs for people with health problems, adaptive exercises, tai chi, yoga, pilates, fitness trails, and others. Check with your local "Y," community center, department of parks and recreation, adult education program, and community college. There is a great deal of variation in the content of these programs, and in the professional experience of the exercise staff. By and large, the classes are inexpensive, and program planners are responsive to people's needs.

Health and fitness clubs usually offer aerobic studios, weight training, cardiovascular equipment, and sometimes a heated pool. For all these services they charge membership fees, which can be high. But some clubs have discounts for people with HIV/AIDS. Ask about low-impact and beginners' exercise classes, both in the aerobic studio and in the pool.* Gyms that emphasize weight lifting exclusively generally don't have the programs or personnel to help you with a flexible, overall fitness program.

In choosing an exercise class or health and fitness club, look for the following qualities:

- Classes designed for *moderate- and low-intensity* exercise. You should be able to observe classes and participate in at least one class before signing up and paying.

---

* You may be wondering whether it's safe for others if you use a public pool or exercise/fitness equipment. Are you putting other people at risk for catching HIV from you? Let's be clear here, because we don't want you avoiding exercise out of concern for others: *It is not dangerous for you to use public pools or exercise equipment or to play group sports.* No one has ever caught HIV from any kind of group sport or exercise. So just use common sense. If you're bleeding, stop your exercise and clean up after yourself. All people should do the same, whether they have HIV or not.

- Instructors with *qualifications and experience.* Knowledgeable instructors are more likely to understand special needs and be willing and able to work with you. Being knowledgeable means knowing not only about exercise but also something about working with people with HIV/AIDS.

- Membership policies that allow you to pay for only a session of classes, or let you "freeze" membership at times when you can't participate. Some fitness facilities offer *different rates* depending on how many services you use.

- Facilities that are *easy to get to, park near, and enter.* Dressing rooms and exercise sites should be accessible and safe, with professional staff on site.

- A pool that allows *"free swim"* times when the water isn't crowded. Also, find out the policy about children in the pool; small children playing and making noise may not be compatible with your program.

- Staff and other members whom you feel *comfortable* being around.

One last note: There are many excellent videotapes and DVDs for home use. They vary in intensity from very gentle chair exercises to more strenuous aerobic exercise. Ask your doctor, physical therapist, or volunteer agency for suggestions, or review the tapes or discs yourself.

MAINTAINING YOUR COMMITMENT TO EXERCISE

If you haven't exercised recently, you'll undoubtedly experience some new feelings and discomfort in the early days of your fitness program. Most of these new feelings are normal and expected, but a few may mean you should change what you're doing. See "Advice for Exercise Problems" on page 215 if you're concerned. Remember, it's normal to feel muscle tension and tenderness around joints and to be a little more tired in the evenings. *Muscle or joint pain that lasts more than two hours after the exercise, or feeling tired into the next day, means that you probably did too much too fast. Don't stop;* just exercise less vigorously or for a shorter time the next day.

IMPLEMENTING A SUCCESSFUL FITNESS PROGRAM

- Keep your exercise goal in mind.

- Choose exercises you want to do. Combine activities that move you toward your goal and are recommended by your health care providers.

- Choose the time and place to exercise. Tell your partner, family, and friends your plan.

- Make an action plan for yourself. Decide how long you'll stick with these particular exercises. Six to eight weeks is a reasonable time commitment for a new program.

- Try keeping an exercise diary or calendar, leaving space to write down your exercises, how long you do them, your heart rate or perceived exertion score, and your feelings before and after exercise. Put your diary where you can see it, and fill it out every day.

- Do some self-tests to keep track of your progress. Distance and time self-tests appear on pages 207–208. Record the date and results. You may also use your exercise diary for this purpose.

- Start your program. Remember to begin gradually and proceed slowly, especially if you haven't exercised in a while.

- Repeat the self-tests at regular intervals, record the results, and check the changes.

- Revise your program. At the end of six to eight weeks, decide what you liked, what worked, and what made exercising difficult. Modify your program and make another action plan for the next few weeks. You may decide to change some of the exercises, the place or time that you exercise, or your exercise partners.

- Reward yourself for a job well done. Many people who start an exercise program find that the rewards come with improved fitness and endurance. Being able to enjoy outings, a refreshing walk, or trips to a store, the library, a concert, or a museum are great rewards to look forward to.

When you do aerobic exercise, it's natural to feel your heart beat faster, your breathing speed up, and your body get warmer. However, irregular or very rapid heartbeats, excessive shortness of breath, or dizziness are not what you want. If this happens to you, stop exercising and discontinue your program until you check with your doctor.

If you have symptoms such as fatigue, shortness of breath, or physical discomfort, it can be difficult at first to figure out whether these are caused by the illness, medication, exercise, or some combination of these. Talking to someone else with HIV/AIDS about his or her experience in starting an exercise program may help. Once you are able to sort out some of these sensations, you'll be able to exercise with confidence.

Expect setbacks. During the first year of an exercise program, people average two to three interruptions in their exercise schedule, often because of minor injuries or illnesses unrelated to their exercise. You may find yourself sidelined or derailed temporarily. Don't be discouraged. Try a different activity or simply rest. When you are feeling better, resume your program, but begin at a lower, more gentle level. As a rule of thumb, it will take you the same amount of time to get back into shape as you were out. For instance, if you missed three weeks, it may take at least three weeks to get back to your previous level. Go slowly. Be kind to yourself. You're in this for the long haul.

Think of your head as the coach and your body as the team. For success, all parts of your team need attention. Be a good coach. *Encourage and praise yourself.* Design "plays" you feel your team can execute successfully. Choose places that are safe and hospitable. A good coach knows his or her team, sets good goals, and helps the team succeed. A good coach is loyal. A good coach does not belittle, nag, or make anyone feel guilty. Be a good coach.

Besides a good coach, everyone needs an enthusiastic cheerleader or two. Of course, you can be your own cheerleader, but being both coach and cheerleader is a lot to do. A successful exerciser usually has at least one *family member or close friend who actively supports* his or her exercise program. Your cheerleader can exercise with you, help you get chores done so you have time to exercise, praise your accomplishments, or just take your exercise time into consideration when making plans. Sometimes cheerleaders pop up by themselves, but don't be bashful about asking for a hand.

ADVICE FOR EXERCISE PROBLEMS

Problem	Advice
Irregular or very rapid heartbeat	Stop exercising. Check your pulse. Are the beats regular or irregular? How fast is your heartbeat? Make a note of this information, and discuss it with your doctor before exercising again.
Pain, tightness, or pressure in your chest, jaw, arms, neck, or back	Stop exercising and sit or lie down. If the pain, tightness, or pressure lasts more than fifteen minutes, go to an emergency department AT ONCE! Don't wait. Check with your doctor about these symptoms before exercising again.
Unusual, extreme shortness of breath, persisting ten minutes after you exercise	Notify your doctor and get clearance before exercising again.
Lightheadedness, dizziness, fainting, cold sweat, or confusion	Lie down with your feet up, or sit down and put your head between your legs. If it happens more than once, check with your doctor before exercising again.
Excessive tiredness after exercise, especially if you're still tired twenty-five hours after you exercise	Don't exercise so vigorously next time. If the excessive tiredness persists, check with your doctor.

With exercise experience, you develop a sense of control in your life. You learn how to *alternate your activities to fit your day-to-day needs.* You know when to do less and when to do more. You know that a change in symptoms or a period of inactivity are usually only temporary and don't have to be devastating. You know you have the tools to get back on track again.

Give your exercise plan a chance to succeed. Set reasonable goals and enjoy your success. Stay motivated. When it comes to your personal fitness program, sticking with it and doing it your way make you a definite winner.

EXERCISE RESOURCES

- Adult education
- Hospitals, health care organizations
- Community colleges
- Parks and recreation programs
- Health and fitness clubs
- YMCA, YWCA

SUGGESTED READING

Ciccolo, J. T., Jowers, E. M., and Bartholomew, J. B. "The Benefits of Exercise Training for Quality of Life in HIV/AIDS in the Post-HAART Era" in *Sports Medicine* 34 (8): 487–499, 2004.

Cooper, Kenneth H. *Overcoming Hypertension: Dr. Kenneth Cooper's Preventive Medicine Program.* New York: Bantam Doubleday, 1991.

Exercise and Physical Fitness at Medline Plus Web site. http://www. nlm.nih.gov/medlineplus/exerciseandphysicalfitness.html. Accessed August 10, 2005.

Huey, Lynda, and Forster, Robert. *The Complete Waterpower Workout Book: Programs for Fitness, Injury Prevention, and Healing.* New York: Random House, 1993.

Klemack, C. *Benefits of Exercise for People with HIV/AIDS.* The National Center on Physical Activity and Disability at http://www.ncpad.org/disability/. Accessed August 10, 2005.

Nixon, S., O'Brien, K., Glazier, R. H., and Tynan, A. M. "Aerobic Exercise Interventions for Adults Living with HIV/AIDS" in *The Cochrane Database of Systematic Reviews.* 2005, Issue 2. Art. No.: CD001796.pub2.DOI:10.1002/14651858.CD001796.pub2.

Sayce, Valerie, and Frasier, Ian. *Exercise Beats Arthritis: An Easy-to-Follow Program of Exercises.* Boulder, Colo.: Bull Publishing, 1998, and Melbourne, Australia: Frasier Publications, 1987.

Stewart, Gordon W. *Active Living: The Miracle Medicine for a Long and Healthy Life.* Champaign, Ill.: Human Kinetics, 1995.

Van Fulpen, Charles D. *Guide to Contented Hearts: Cardiac Risk Management: Cholesterol, High Blood Pressure, Exercise, Stress, Weight, Diet.* Kalamazoo, Mich.: Contented Hearts, Inc. 1995.

Vedral, Joyce L. *Bone Building Body Shaping Workout: Strength, Health, Beauty in Just 16 Minutes a Day.* New York: Fireside, 1998.

White, Martha. *Water Exercise: 78 Safe and Effective Exercises for Fitness and Therapy.* Champaign, Ill.: Human Kinetics, 1995.

CHAPTER TWELVE

Healthy Eating

Eating healthy foods is important for everyone, and a healthy diet is a valuable tool for HIV/AIDS management. A nutritionally balanced eating plan gives you more energy and strength to carry out your daily activities and enjoy life as much as possible. It also helps your body's immune system to fight off infections, and can control or even prevent other health problems. Although there is currently no cure for HIV/AIDS, we do know that healthy eating helps to slow the disease process, prevent weight loss, lower blood sugar and cholesterol levels, and control some of the unpleasant side effects of medications, thereby contributing to your quality of life.

In this chapter we offer some guidelines to consider when developing a healthy eating plan. We also discuss ways to manage some of the common eating problems associated with HIV disease and medication side effects, and how to manage health problems such as diabetes and heart disease that may develop with HIV treatments. In Chapter 13, we provide important tips on food safety and preparation. Just as with the other self-management techniques discussed in this book, putting these suggestions into practice can help you feel more in control of your health and your life.

WHAT IS HEALTHY EATING?

Healthy eating means choosing healthier foods, finding better ways to prepare these foods, and eating in moderation. For people with HIV/AIDS, however, figuring out what foods to eat becomes a challenge because disease symptoms and/or medications can interfere with the ability or desire to eat. Although there is no one answer for every person, these general guideline may help:

- *Eat a variety of healthy foods in appropriate amounts regularly throughout the day.* The specific amounts of these foods and how many times a day you eat will vary depending on your individual health condition, nutritional needs, and eating challenges. To establish your own eating plan, it helps to keep a few basic principles in mind. See "Principles of Healthy Eating," page 222.

- *Eating a variety of foods from the different food groups every day* helps you get all the nutrients your body needs to function well. These nutrients include protein, carbohydrates, fats, vitamins, minerals, and water. Each nutrient plays an important role in your body. Unfortunately, no one food contains them all; therefore, we must eat a variety of foods from different groups. To see which foods contain these necessary nutrients, refer to "Essential Nutrients, Their Functions, and Food Sources," page 229.

- *Eating small, frequent meals or snacks at regular times throughout the day* provides you with the energy needed to maintain your bodily functions and muscle weight. It also helps your body absorb and use medications, and it lessens some of the medications' side effects. For people with health concerns such as diabetes, infections, chronic diarrhea, and weight problems, it is especially important to eat small, frequent meals. For example, with diabetes, how much and when you eat affects your blood sugar levels. Watching the size of portions, spreading your meals out over four- to five-hour intervals, and not skipping meals all help to keep your blood sugar within an appropriate range. If you have been losing weight because you have little or no appetite or are fighting off an infection or other illness, you may need to modify your eating plan to include more protein and/or calories as well as vitamins and minerals. See "Getting More Calories and Protein," page 244. You may also consider talking with your doctor or a nutritionist about other ways to adjust your eating plan to meet your specific health needs and lifestyle.

- *Eating the same amount at each meal* ensures that your body has an adequate supply of energy to function at an optimal level during the day. Not eating enough or skipping meals can throw your system off and lead to snacking on sweets or fast and easy "junk" foods that are higher in fat and sugar. Skipping meals can also aggravate symptoms or cause other problems, such as irritability, mood swings, and low blood sugar. Eating too much at one meal causes problems, too, such as indigestion, discomfort, and difficulties with breathing. Eating too much can also contribute to weight gain and poor sleep.

- *Increasing the amount of protein and calories you eat* is important if you are having difficulty maintaining your weight. If you have trouble eating food, try drinking high-calorie fluids (juices, nectars, Gatorade) or high-protein drinks (milk, milk shakes, fortified milk, soy milk, Ensure Plus, Nutren 2.0, Nutrament, Resource Plus, Sustacal) in place of or in addition to water.

- *Reducing or limiting the amount of carbohydrates, fats, and cholesterol you eat at each meal will help to prevent or control diabetes and heart disease.* For people with diabetes, it is important to limit carbohydrates in order to help control blood sugar levels. The recommended amount of carbohydrates for each regular meal is between forty-five and sixty grams. The food guide on pages 223–227 lists some foods that provide carbohydrates, and recommends portion sizes to help you get the right amount of carbohydrates at each meal.

- *For people at risk for heart disease, it is important to eat less fat and cholesterol and increase fiber intake.* This helps prevent the narrowing and hardening of the arteries that can cause heart attacks. Reducing fat also helps with weight and blood pressure control. The food guide shows the fat and cholesterol content of different foods, and lists some fatty foods to avoid. See "Hints for Reducing Fat in Your Eating Plan," page 252, and "Hints for Increasing Fiber in Your Eating Plan," on page 253.

- *Drinking plenty of fluids every day* is vital, especially if you are taking medications. Your body needs water in order to function normally, to use nutrients and medications efficiently, and to eliminate waste and toxins. Because the body uses water to help flush out medications, you must take in more fluid to prevent dehydration. You should drink at least eight full glasses of water and other liquids each day. If you are taking many medications, drink more liquid. Try to avoid drinks that contain caffeine (coffee, some dark teas, and some sodas) or alcohol; these types of drinks are low in nutrients.

PRINCIPLES OF HEALTHY EATING

Eat a variety of foods from each food group every day.

Eat small, frequent meals or have snacks at regular intervals during the day.

Eat the same amount of food at each meal.

Increase the amount of protein and calories you eat if your weight is below normal, if you are not eating enough, or if you have chronic diarrhea.

Reduce or limit the amount of carbohydrates, fats, and cholesterol you eat at each meal, to help prevent or control diabetes and heart disease. This is especially important if you have lipodystrophy or are taking HAART medications.

Drink plenty of fluids each day (at least eight full glasses).

Take a multivitamin/mineral supplement every day.

Avoid chemical stimulants, such as:

- Caffeine (coffee, some dark teas, regular sodas)

- Alcoholic drinks (beer, wine, and liquor)

- Recreational drugs (cigarettes, cigars, cocaine, marijuana, "speed," etc.)

FOOD GUIDE FORMULA FOR HEALTHY EATING

One portion of PROTEINS + one portion of VEGETABLES + one portion of
FRUIT + two portions of STARCH/CARBOHYDRATES

PROTEINS: One portion exchange = proteins, fats, and carbohydrates

	Portion		Portion
CHEESE: *(0 g carbohydrates, 7 g protein per oz; grams fat varies)*		**MEATS:** *(0 g carbohydrates, 7 g protein per oz)*	
Fresh (Mexican) cheese	2–3 oz	Lean 0–3 g fat per oz: round, sirloin, flank, tenderloin	2–3 oz
Cottage cheese (low-fat)	¼ cup	Medium-fat 5 g fat per oz: ground beef, corned beef, prime rib	2–3 oz
Regular cheese (8 g fat per oz)	2–3 oz	High-fat 8 g fat per oz: spare rib, ground pork, pork sausage	2–3 oz
MILK: *(12 g carbohydrates, 8 g protein; grams fat varies)*		**POULTRY: chicken, turkey, hen** *(0 g carbohydrates, 7 g protein per oz)*	
Milk, nonfat, low fat	1 cup	Lean 0–3 g fat: white meat, skinless breast	2–3 oz
Powdered milk	1 tbsp	Medium-fat 5 g fat: dark meat, leg or thigh/skin	2–3 oz
Whole milk	1 cup	High-fat 8 g fat: fried chicken/skin, duck	2–3 oz
Soy milk	1 cup		
YOGURT: *(20 g carbohydrates, 8 g protein)*		**PROCESSED MEAT/LUNCH MEAT:**	
Yogurt (low fat, varies)	1 cup	Low-fat: turkey, ham, beef, hot dogs, hamburger meat *(high in sodium)*	2–3 oz
EGGS: *(0 g carbohydrates, 7 g protein)*		**ORGAN MEATS:** *(high in cholesterol)*	
Fresh eggs *(high in cholesterol)*	1 egg	Liver, tripe, brains, tongue, etc.	2–3 oz
Note: Meat portions measured by the size of the palm of your hand and ½ to 1 inch (1 to 2 cm) thickness		**OTHER:**	
FISH: *(0 g carbohydrates, 7 g protein per oz)*		Tofu *(0 g carbohydrates, 7 g protein, 3 g fat)*	½ cup
Lean 0–3 g fat per oz: Cod, halibut, flounder, haddock, trout, tuna, salmon, sardines, oysters on the half shell, shrimp	2–3 oz	Peanut butter *(0 g carbohydrates, 7 g protein, 8 g fat)*	2 tbsp
Medium-fat 5 g fat per oz: Any fried fish	2–3 oz		

CONTINUED ON NEXT PAGE

FOOD GUIDE FORMULA FOR HEALTHY EATING (CONTINUED)

VEGETABLES LOW IN STARCH

	Portion		Portion
Vegetables low in starch can be eaten as often as you like.		Green onion or scallions	
Fresh, Frozen or Canned (low-sodium)*		Nopales (cactus)	
Artichoke		Mushrooms	
Asparagus		Okra	
Broccoli		Onions	
Brussel sprouts		Peppers (red and green)	
Bean sprouts		Radish	
Cabbage, Chinese cabbage		Salad greens	
Celery		Squash	
Chayote (vegetable pear)		Spinach	
Chicory		Tomato	
Chilies, spicy		Turnips	
Cucumber		Watercress	
Cauliflower		Zucchini	
Eggplant (aubergine)		**Vegetable Juices**	
Garlic		Mixed vegetables (V-8)	½ cup
Green beans		Tomato	¼ cup

FREE FOOD LIST:
(Contains less than 5 g of carbohydrates per serving)

DRINKS		**DRINKS (continued)**	
Atol (cornmeal drink)	1 cup	Coffee	
Bouillion or broth (chicken or beef)		Diet soft drinks, sugar-free	1 cup
		Drink mixes, sugar-free	
Bouillion or broth, low-sodium	1 cup	Horchata (rice drink)	½ cup
Carbonated or mineral water		Tea	
Club soda		Tonic water, sugar-free	
Cocoa powder (3 tsp)	1 cup		

* Foods listed without a serving size can be eaten as often as you like

CONTINUED ON NEXT PAGE

FOOD GUIDE FORMULA FOR HEALTHY EATING (CONTINUED)

STARCHY VEGETABLES: One portion exchange = 15 g carbohydrate, 3–7 g protein, 0–1 g fat (if oil added)

	Portion		Portion
Beans, lentils, peas	½ cup	Snow peas	½ cup
Beets	½ cup	Squash, winter	½ cup
Carrots	½ cup	Yam, sweet potato	½ cup
Corn	½ cup	Yautia	½ cup
Jicama	½ cup		
Plantain	½ cup		
Potato, baked or boiled	1 cup		

STARCH/CARBOHYDRATES:
One portion exchange = 15 g carbohydrate, 3 g protein, 0–1 g fat

PASTA, CEREALS AND GRAINS

Bran cereals	½ cup
Cereals, unsweetened	¾ cup
Granola, low-fat	¼ cup
Oats, plain	½ cup
Rice Krispies	½ cup
Wheat germ	3 tbsp
Pasta	½ cup
Rice, cooked	½ cup

BREAD

Roll, regular	½
White, whole wheat	1 slice
Bread (made of milk/salt, small)	½
English muffin, plain	½
Hot dog or hamburger bun	½
Pancake, regular, low-fat	1
Pita bread, 6 inches across	½
Tortilla, corn, regular	1
Tortilla, flour, medium	1
Waffle, regular, low-fat	1

FATS:
One portion exchange = 5 g fat

MONOUNSATURATED FAT

Avocado, medium	¼
Nuts:	
almonds, cashews	6 nuts
peanuts	8 nuts
pecans, walnuts	4 halves

Peanut butter, crunchy	2 tbsp
Olives, all types (large)	5
Sesame seeds	1 tsp

CONTINUED ON NEXT PAGE

FOOD GUIDE FORMULA FOR HEALTHY EATING (CONTINUED)

FRUITS:
One portion exchange = 15 g carbohydrate

	Portion		Portion
Fresh		Peach, medium	1
Apple, small	1	Plum, small	1
Apricots, medium	2	Tangerine, medium	1
Banana, small	½	Watermelon	½ cup
Berries: strawberries, blueberries	1 cup	**Canned Fruit**	
Coconut, fresh (shredded)	½ cup	Low-fat/low-sugar	½ cup
Dates	3	Regular	¼ cup
Figs, large	2	**Dried Fruit**	
Grapefruit, small	½ cup	Figs, apricots	2
Grapes, small	½ cup	Raisins	2 tbsp
Guava, medium	2	**Fruit Juices (sugar-free, or low in sugar)**	
Kiwi, large	1	Apple	½ cup
Lemon, large	1	Apricot nectar	½ cup
Lime, large	1	Carbonated juice drinks	½ cup
Mango, small	1	Fruit punch	½ cup
Melon, honeydew	¼	Grapefruit	½ cup
Orange, small	1	Orange	½ cup
Papaya, small	¼	Sweet juices (low in sugar)	½ cup
Pineapple	½ cup	Tamarindo	½ cup
Pear, small	1		
Persimmon, medium	1		

PROBLEM FOODS: Some fats can raise blood cholesterol levels and artificial sugars raise glucose levels

POLYUNSATURATED FATS		SATURATED FATS	
Margarine, low fat	1 tsp	Bacon	1 slice
Mayonnaise, regular	1 tsp	Butter, regular	1 tsp
Mayonnaise, reduced fat	1 tsp	Butter, reduced fat	1 tbsp
Miracle Whip	1 tbsp	Coconut, sweetened (shredded)	2 tbsp
Oil (corn, safflower, soybean)	1 tsp	Cream, half-and-half	2 tbsp
Salad dressing	1 tbsp	Sour cream, regular	2 tbsp
Seeds (pumpkin, sunflower)	1 tsp	Sour cream, reduced fat	3 tbsp
		Shortening or lard	2 tbsp

CONTINUED ON NEXT PAGE

FOOD GUIDE FORMULA FOR HEALTHY EATING (CONTINUED)

PROBLEM FOODS: Some fats can raise blood cholesterol levels and sugars raise glucose levels

	Portion		Portion
DESSERTS, SWEETS		Syrup (sugar-free)	2 tbsp
Cake with frosting	1 slice	Tamal, small	1
Danish, small	1		
Flan, with milk	½ cup	**ALCOHOLIC BEVERAGES**	
Fruit tart or pie	1 slice	Beer	12 oz
Honey	1 tbsp	Champagne	4 oz
Jam or jelly (low-sugar or light)	2 tbsp	Liquor	1 oz
Rice pudding	½ cup	Wine	4 oz

FREE FOOD LIST:
Contains less than 5 g of carbohydrates per serving

SUGAR-FREE FOODS		Gum (sugar-free)
Candy, hard (sugar-free)	1 candy	Sugar substitutes
Gelatin dessert (sugar-free)		
Gelatin, unflavored		

Recommendations:

+ Recommended portion of sodium is 400 mg

* Foods listed without a serving size can be eaten as often as you like

• Sugar substitutes, alternatives, or replacements that are approved by the Food and Drug Administration (FDA) are safe to use. Common brand names include: Equal® (aspartame); Sweet One® (acesulfame K); Sugar Twin® (saccharin); Sprinkle Sweet® (saccharin); Sweet-10® (saccharin); Sweet 'n' Low® (saccharin)

Abbreviations for the measurement units:

Grams	g	Tablespoon	tbsp
Teaspoon	tsp	Ounce	oz
Milligrams	mg		

A Word About Water and Vitamin and Mineral Supplements

There are elements of a healthy diet that are not food. Besides eating right, it is important to make good choices about the water you drink and the supplements you take.

Because some germs can be spread through tap water, it is better to drink bottled water. This can be distilled water, spring water filtered to two microns, or carbonated soda water. If you want to use tap water to drink or to make ice cubes or juices, boil the water for at least five minutes. If you drink bottled juices, choose those that are pasteurized, to avoid bacteria that can make you sick. This is especially important when your immune system is suppressed.

You may benefit from *taking daily multivitamin and mineral supplements.* Deficiencies in vitamins A, B6, and C, and in minerals such as zinc, selenium, iron, and copper can worsen the immune suppression caused by not eating enough protein and calories.

If you are HIV positive and asymptomatic, it is a good idea to take a multivitamin and mineral supplement that provides one hundred percent of the U.S. recommended dietary allowance (RDA) daily. The RDA is a standard level set by the government that has been determined to prevent deficiencies and maintain health.

If you are symptomatic, it is a good idea to take two supplement pills (two hundred percent of the RDA) daily with your meals. Research shows that as HIV/AIDS progresses, you can become deficient in other vitamins or minerals (such as vitamin B12 and folate). To determine whether you need higher doses of certain vitamins and minerals, ask your doctor to check your blood levels when you have your regular blood work done.

Many people choose to take therapeutic doses of vitamins and minerals (such as beta-carotene, vitamin E, and vitamin C) to prevent deficiencies and enhance the body's immune function. If you decide to begin taking therapeutic doses of vitamins and minerals, discuss this with your doctor. High doses or overdoses of certain vitamins and minerals (particularly vitamins A, D, and B6; and zinc, selenium, iron, and copper) can cause serious side effects, such as nausea, diarrhea, and loss of appetite; they can even

ESSENTIAL NUTRIENTS, THEIR FUNCTIONS, AND FOOD SOURCES		
Nutrient	**Functions**	**Food Sources**
Proteins	• Build and repair muscle and organ tissues • Build enzymes and hormones • Fight infection • Maintain the body's immune system • Provide energy	Animal sources include meat, fish, poultry, eggs, and dairy products. These provide complete proteins. Vegetable sources, such as legumes (beans and peas), grains, cereals, nuts, seeds, tofu, and soy products are incomplete proteins. These must be eaten together in the right combinations to make complete proteins. They provide fiber and contain no saturated fat.
Carbohydrates	• Provide the major source of energy for the body's metabolism and muscles • Help build and maintain muscles	Starches or complex carbohydrates include grains, rice, pasta, breads, cereals, legumes, (peas and beans), and vegetables. Sugars or simple carbohydrates include fruits and some dairy products. Other simple sugars, such as table sugar, honey,

CONTINUED ON NEXT PAGE

ESSENTIAL NUTRIENTS, THEIR FUNCTIONS, AND FOOD SOURCES		
Nutrient	**Functions**	**Food Sources**
Carbohydrates		syrups, and jellies provide extra calories but have little or no nutritional value.
Fats	• Build body fat and provide extra energy to burn • Help build, strengthen, and repair tissues • Lead to weight gain if eaten in excess	Meat, whole-milk dairy products, nuts, peanuts, seeds, oils, salad dressings, and processed food such as cakes and candies. Eat only moderate amounts of fats—especially saturated fats, which come from animal sources.
Vitamins & Minerals	• Help build strong bones and muscles • Are involved in specific reactions in the body that help it function	These are found in varying amounts in all the different food groups, and interact with other nutrients in the body. Multivitamin and mineral supplements may be necessary if you are HIV positive, because your body may need more of these nutrients than provided in food, especially if you have a poor appetite, skip meals, are fighting off infection, or have chronic diarrhea.

CONTINUED ON NEXT PAGE

ESSENTIAL NUTRIENTS, THEIR FUNCTIONS, AND FOOD SOURCES		
Nutrient	**Functions**	**Food Sources**
Water	• Helps dissolve nutrients and carries them to all parts of the body to be used as energy • Flushes out the body's toxins and waste products • Prevents dehydration and lessens some medication side effects (e.g., dry mouth and constipation)	All foods contain water. Major sources include broth, ice pops, and gelatin. Avoid drinks with caffeine or alcohol, which increase water loss by stimulating urination and causing diarrhea.

damage your liver and kidneys. Taking more than the recommended dose of vitamins and minerals is considered a type of drug therapy, and therefore should be supervised by your physician.

Good brands of over-the-counter (nonprescription) supplements include Centrum and Theragran-M, but there are many others. You may also ask your doctor to write a prescription for a multivitamin and mineral supplement that is covered by the Veterans' Administration, Medicaid, or your state's AIDS Drug Assistance Program (ADAP). If you are considering prescription rather than over-the-counter supplements and are planning to take doses higher than the recommended daily allowance, find out if this is covered by your insurance. (As of this writing, such higher doses are not covered, which means you must pay the costs yourself.)

MAKING A HEALTHY EATING PLAN

Designing and following a healthy eating plan can be difficult. After all, it may involve changing eating habits that you have had for many years. Changing what you eat, how you prepare your food, and how often you eat are not easy things to do, especially if you try to do them all at once. Therefore, to be successful, it is helpful to break your goal into smaller, more manageable steps. This is the essence of being a self-manager.

Step 1: Identify Why You Want to Change Your Eating Plan

This will help motivate you to get started and to stick with the changes you want or need to make. The reasons for changing eating habits differ for each individual. If you have HIV/AIDS, the most obvious reason is to maintain your physical health, but you may also have psychological or emotional reasons for wanting to change. Determine for yourself why you want to make changes. For example, you may want to:

- Lessen disease symptoms or medication side effects

- Lower blood sugar and cholesterol levels to prevent or manage problems such as diabetes and heart disease

- Increase your energy level

- Feel better about yourself

- Strengthen your resistance to infections and other common illnesses

- Change the way others perceive you

- Feel more in control of your disease and your life

If you have other reasons, jot them down below or write them in a journal. You may want to review these periodically to remind yourself of their importance and to help motivate you when you are tempted to give up.

_____

_____

Step 2: Look at What You Eat Now and What You Want or Need to Change

Start by keeping track of what you currently eat. Look at yesterday's meals. Use the food diary on page 000 to list all the foods you ate (including snacks) and the amount or portion size of each. (If you don't want to use this diary, make your own.) If you ate a mixed dish (e.g., pasta with sauce, casserole, or soup), try to estimate how much of each food group was in the serving you ate. Use the portion sizes in the food guide on pages 223–227 to determine the number of servings you had of each food group for the day. Write your total number of servings for the day and compare this to the recommended minimum number of servings for that food group.

You may want to keep a food diary for a few days, including both weekdays and weekends, to help identify your eating patterns. Be sure to note the time of each meal or snack so you can see how frequently you eat. Don't forget to record the fluids you drink during the day. All of this information can help you identify where to start making changes in your eating plan.

Step 3: Decide When and How to Start

Success is important when you are trying something new or making any kind of change. This is especially true when it comes to eating. If you are successful at the beginning, you will be more likely to stick with your new habits, and will be motivated to make more changes as needed. Therefore, it is wise to look ahead to identify the factors that will help you make the changes you want, and the factors that may make it difficult to change. For example, consider the following types of questions:

- Is there someone who will support you, or something you can do to make it easier to change?

- Will worries or concerns about friends, work, or other commitments affect your ability to follow through?

- How can you coordinate your medications with food?

- How will medications affect your appetite?

- Are there obstacles that will keep you from changing the way you eat?

SAMPLE FOOD DIARY			
Time of Meal/Snack	What You Ate	How Much (Portion Size)	Number of Servings for Each Food Group
			__ Protein __Vegetables __ Dairy __Fruit __ Starch __Fats & sweets
			__ Protein __Vegetables __ Dairy __Fruit __ Starch __Fats & sweets
			__ Protein __Vegetables __ Dairy __Fruit __ Starch __Fats & sweets
			__ Protein __Vegetables __ Dairy __Fruit __ Starch __Fats & sweets
			__ Protein __Vegetables __ Dairy __Fruit __ Starch __Fats & sweets
			__ Protein __Vegetables __ Dairy __Fruit __ Starch __Fats & sweets

Examine all these factors. Then find ways to build support for the desired changes or to minimize any problems you anticipate. Once you have done this, set the date on which you will begin making your changes. If it is too difficult to start right now, set a date in the near future to reevaluate your plan. In the meantime, accept that this is the right decision for you, and focus your attention on other goals. You do not have to change everything at once.

When you are ready, begin with the changes that are easiest. Make one change at a time. You may decide to change how often you eat before changing what you eat. If you skip meals now, it may be a good idea to start by eating more regularly. After you get into the habit of eating four or more times a day, you may make other changes, such as adding more vegetables and fruits to your eating plan, or eating more breads and cereals.

Step 4: Put Your New Eating Plan into Practice

This is often the hardest step. Therefore, we provide the "Formula for Healthy Eating" on page 236, and the food guide on pages 223–227, to help you plan and prepare healthier meals and snacks. Our formula not only offers variety in the foods you can eat, but also encourages you to eat more servings of vegetables and fruits (at least five a day) and to choose appropriate portion sizes.

In addition to using these guidelines, it is a good idea to read the nutrition labels on the foods you buy. Most foods have labels that list their nutritional content under the heading, "Nutrition Facts." Usually there are so many facts listed on the label that we either don't understand them or get confused and give up. However, it is useful to understand at least some of the more important facts on these labels if we want to make healthier choices. These include the serving or portion size, number of servings per package, and total carbohydrates, fat, cholesterol, and sodium. "Nutrition Facts to Look for on Food Labels" on page 237 outlines more specifically what to look for. On some packages, the label may be too small to list the nutritional content; by law, however, the manufacturer must provide this information to the consumer. Therefore, there is usually a telephone number, address, and even a Web site to contact for nutrition information.

FORMULA FOR HEALTHY EATING			
Nutrient	Examples of Foods	Recommended Portion/Meal	Total Recommended Amount per Meal
Protein	Meat, fish, poultry, milk products, eggs, beans or peas, nuts or seeds, tofu	1	35 grams total for each meal
Carbohydrates	Vegetables, starches (e.g., breads, cereal rice, pasta), fruit	1 or more 2 1	45–60 grams total
Fats	Meats low in fat, vegetable oils, dressings, milk products, avocado, peanuts	1–3 grams portion	10 grams total for each meal
Sodium	Processed products labeled "low salt"	As little as possible	400 milligrams for each meal

NUTRITION FACTS TO LOOK FOR ON FOOD LABELS

- The serving size and servings per container are important. Many products have more than one serving or portion per package. Also, it is possible that even the amount in one serving is more than what is recommended for certain nutrients. (This example is 1 serving size, and there is 1 serving per container.)

- The amount of total carbohydrates is listed per serving, not per package, which is 39 g in this example. This includes the amount of fiber (2 g) as well as sugars (2 g) in or added to the product. This fact is especially important for individuals watching or counting their carbohydrates.

- The amount of total fat (7 g in this example) includes saturated fat (3.5 g) and unsaturated fat (not listed). For individuals watching their fat intake, the total fat should be 5 grams per serving. Look for products with less saturated fat.

- Be aware of the amount of cholesterol (15 mg in this example). Lower is better. Products with less saturated fat also have less cholesterol.

- Note the amount of sodium (890 mg in this example). The recommended amount is less than 400 mg per serving.

Nutrition Facts

Serving Size 1 Entree (227 g)
Servings Per Container 1

Amount Per Serving

Calories 250   Calories from Fat 60

	% Daily Value*
Total Fat 7 g	11%
Saturated Fat 3.5 g	17%
Cholesterol 15 mg	5%
Sodium 890 mg	37%
Total Carbohydrate 39 g	13%
Dietary Fiber 2 g	8%
Sugars 2 g	
Protein 8 g	

Vitamin A 20%	•	Vitamin C 15%
Calcium 10%	•	Iron 6%

*Percent Daily Values are based on a 2,000 calorie diet.

As you start putting your new eating plan into practice, it may be helpful to make an action plan as discussed in Chapter 2, "Becoming an HIV/AIDS Self-Manager." This will help you incorporate new practices into your daily routine. In addition, the following ideas may help you overcome some of the problems many of us encounter when trying to change our eating habits.

DEALING WITH PROBLEMS IN CHANGING EATING HABITS

I eat out a lot, so how do I know if I'm eating well?

Whether it's because you don't have enough time, hate to cook, or just don't have the energy to go grocery shopping and prepare meals, eating out may suit your needs. This is not necessarily bad, if you know which choices are healthy ones. These tips may help:

- Select restaurants that not only serve a variety of dishes but also offer variety in the way they prepare those dishes. Nowadays many restaurants, including some fast-food chains, offer nutritious food choices. For example, you can choose a dish that is grilled or broiled rather than fried, or a salad and baked potato instead of a hamburger and fries.

- Ask what is in a dish and how it is prepared, especially if it is a dish you have not tried before.

- Choose restaurants that list ingredients on their menus. That way, you can order dishes that are right for your special needs, whether you are trying to increase protein or fiber, reduce fat, add calories, or limit carbohydrates.

- Follow the food safety guidelines for eating out in Chapter 13, "Food Safety and Preparation Tips."

I know some foods are good for me, but I just don't like them.

If you don't like a certain food, try substituting another food in the same food group. If you don't like an entire food group, you may need to consult a nutritionist to find foods from other groups that can give you similar nutrients.

I don't like vegetables.

Try raw vegetables with tasty dips or sauces to add flavor. Grated or frozen vegetables can be added to soups, stews, or meat loaf. Try vegetable casseroles, such as vegetable lasagna. If vegetables still don't appeal to you, increase the amounts of fruits and breads you eat.

I don't like to drink milk.

Instead of drinking milk, add it (or dry milk powder) to foods such as soups, meat loaf, or casseroles. You can also choose pudding, yogurt, cottage cheese, or ice cream in place of milk. Try yogurt in a salad dressing or in a vegetable or fruit dip. Melt some cheese on vegetables, on potatoes, on beans, on tortillas, in sandwiches, on pizza, or in a dip. To get some of the same nutrients that are in milk without eating cheese or yogurt, try broccoli, greens (such as kale or collard or beet greens), tofu, beans, canned salmon, and corn tortillas. If milk or milk products make you feel bloated and cause diarrhea or gas, see the discussion of dairy products and lactose intolerance on page 249.

I'm a vegetarian. I don't want to eat any animal foods.

You can be a vegetarian and still have a healthy eating plan. To make sure you get the protein and other nutrients usually supplied by food from animals, include fortified soybean milk, tofu, beans, and other plant protein sources along with a variety of breads, grains, pasta, fruits, and vegetables. If meat, fish, and poultry are the only animal foods you don't eat, include a variety of dairy products and eggs.

I eat when I'm feeling bored, depressed, lonely, or otherwise discontent.

Many people find comfort in food. Some people eat when they don't have anything else to do. Some eat when they're feeling "down" or bothered. Unfortunately, at these times you may lose track of what and how much you eat. These are also times when "healthy" foods, such as fruits and vegetables, just don't satisfy your hunger urge. The following strategies can help:

- Keep track of your eating patterns. List what, how much, and when you eat. Note how you are feeling (bored, frustrated, sad) when you have the urge to eat. Try to spot patterns.

- Make a plan for when these situations arise. If you catch yourself feeling bored or down in the dumps, try to do something else instead of eating "junk" food. Do some light exercise, practice a relaxation or distraction technique, or engage in your favorite hobby.

I'd rather eat sweets and snack foods such as chips, candy, and cookies.

You can include these foods in your meals and snacks; in fact, they can be important sources of calories. But try to eat foods from each of the primary food groups first. If you're still hungry or if you have a taste for more, then add moderate portions of your favorite sweets and snack foods. Try not to let chips, candy, and cookies take the place of other foods that are more nutritious.

It takes too long to prepare meals. By the time I'm done, I'm too tired to eat!

You need to eat to maintain your energy level. If meal preparation is a problem for you, it's time to develop a plan. Here are some energy-saving suggestions:

- Plan your meals for the week. Then go to the grocery store and buy everything you will need.

- Break your food preparation into steps, resting in between.

- Cook enough for two, three, or even more servings, especially if it's something you really like.

- Freeze the extra portions in single-serving sizes. On days when you are really tired, thaw and reheat one of these precooked frozen meals.

- Ask for help, especially for big meals or at social gatherings.

I've never really been a cook, and I can't start now.

Keep it simple. Keep your freezer stocked with prepared meals: pizzas, vegetables, and other convenience foods. Try easy-to-prepare meals such as a grilled cheese sandwich and canned soup, eggs and toast, cereal and milk, or macaroni and cheese. Go to the library or a bookstore and look through some cookbooks to get ideas for quick meals. When you do cook, make larger amounts and freeze portions to reheat later.

MANAGING SPECIFIC EATING PROBLEMS

Like everyone, you want to eat healthy food that tastes good and makes you feel good. But having HIV/AIDS may create specific eating problems that are not common in other people. The symptoms you experience from an infection, from depression, or as medication side effects often affect how you feel about eating. The result can be weight loss, which weakens the body's ability to fight off other illnesses. Some medications can cause other conditions, such as high cholesterol and high blood sugar (hyperglycemia or even diabetes), which may require even more changes in your eating plan. Eating a variety of foods and maintaining a healthy weight are important goals for the person with HIV; therefore, it is necessary to find ways to deal with some of the specific problems that interfere with your eating. Let's look at some of these problems.

I don't feel like eating anything.

Loss of appetite is a common problem that can be caused by medication, fatigue, concern about your illness, or an infection. On days when you feel like eating, be sure to eat plenty to make up for days when your appetite is poor. When you are having trouble with appetite, the following suggestions can help you get the calories you need.

- Eat smaller meals more frequently (six times a day).

- Eat in a relaxed setting, with a friend, or while listening to your favorite music.

- Keep food by your bed so you can eat something if you wake at night.

- Eat your favorite foods as often as you like, even if in small amounts.

- Add more flavor to your foods with spices and herbs, lemon wedges, mustard, barbecue sauce, catsup, or hot sauce.

- Have take-out food delivered to your home, or check in your area for home food-delivery services, such as Project Open Hand or Meals on Wheels.

- Keep a supply of high-calorie, high-protein snacks on hand, such as crackers, cheese, peanut butter, and ice cream. Eat these whenever you feel like it.

- Try liquid foods or foods that do not take a lot of energy to chew or cook. When you don't feel like eating much, make a milk shake or have a supplement drink. (Your doctor, nurse, or nutritionist can recommend one.)

- Avoid filling up on liquids before you eat. Drink small amounts when you eat, and sip fluids between your eating times.

- Keep easy-to-prepare foods on hand, such as canned food, frozen meals, or frozen leftovers.

- Pack nonperishable food to snack on when you are away from home. Keep snacks in handy places around the house—for example, near your bedside or where you relax at home.

- Do light exercise before you eat to help increase your appetite.

- Ask your doctor about medications or natural remedies that can stimulate your appetite, especially if you seem to be losing weight.

It's important to eat enough calories and nutrients to avoid weight loss. If you find that you can't keep your appetite up, consult your doctor. He or she can refer you to a nutritionist, who can help you plan meals that maximize the value of what you eat.

I get full too fast.

Eat often during the day. Three meals a day may not be enough for you, especially if you can't eat a full meal at one sitting. Eating five or six times per day seems to work best for most people with HIV/AIDS, particularly those who do not feel well. Make what you eat count: Choose foods with lots of calories and protein to help meet your needs for these important nutrients. (See "Getting More Calories and Protein," page 244.)

Food doesn't taste as good as before.

Mouth infections, such as thrush, and certain medications can change your taste sensations and ability to enjoy food. You may also experience a bitter or metallic taste in your mouth. The following suggestions can help you manage this problem and enhance the flavor of food:

- Rinse your mouth with a mixture of one teaspoon of hydrogen peroxide or baking soda in a glass of warm distilled water before eating. Swish the mixture around in your mouth, but do not swallow. Also, if oral or esophageal thrush is a problem for you, remember to take your antifungal medication to prevent it.

- Use flavored toothpaste on a soft-bristled toothbrush to clean your teeth and tongue before and after you eat.

- To mask the metallic taste, try drinking orange, cranberry, or pineapple juice; lemonade; or another tart drink.

- Marinate meat, poultry, fish, or tofu in vinegar, wine, salad dressing, or soy sauce.

- Eat cold foods such as sherbet, fruit ice, frozen yogurt, and ice cream to numb your taste buds.

- Chew your food well so that it will remain in your mouth longer to stimulate your taste buds.

Modify recipes to include a variety of ingredients that make your food look and taste more appealing. Add vinegar, lemon juice, pickles, or fresh and dried herbs to your food. Start with about one-quarter teaspoon of herbs (rosemary, thyme, basil, oregano, cilantro, cumin) in a dish that serves four. Try adding chopped nuts or seeds to your food; this gives the food a different texture and makes eating a bit more interesting.

Getting More Calories and Protein	
Add:	**To:**
Butter, margarine, sour cream	Vegetables, cooked cereal, potatoes, noodles, or rice
Dried fruits or nuts, honey, jelly, jam, syrup, sugar, cream, half-and-half, yogurt	Hot or cold cereal, pancakes, or waffles
Bacon, avocado, olives, mayonnaise, salad dressing	Sandwiches, salads, or casseroles
Cream or sour cream	Soups, fruit, or puddings
Cheese or cream cheese	Fruit or crackers
Peanut butter or other nut butter	Sauces, shakes, toast, crackers, waffles, fresh fruit, or raw vegetables
Chopped meat; canned tuna, salmon, shrimp, or crab meat; shredded cheese; hard-cooked eggs; egg substitutes; beans; tofu	Soups, sauces, vegetables, salads, or casseroles
Gravy	Meat, poultry, or potatoes
Honey, sugar, molasses, syrup	Milk shakes, hot or cold tea, Kool-Aid, or lemonade
Dried fruit, syrup	Ice cream, yogurt, or frozen yogurt
Powdered milk	Regular milk, scrambled eggs, soups, gravies, or desserts

When I eat, I feel like I'm going to throw up.

An infection or a medication side effect can cause nausea, making foods unappealing. The following suggestions may help you to manage these symptoms:

- Eat smaller, snack-sized meals throughout the day. Nausea is often worse when the stomach is empty

- Drink high-calorie fluids one hour after eating, not during meals.

- Avoid spicy and fatty foods and caffeine. These can irritate the stomach and intestines.

- Eat cold, blander-tasting foods such as ice cream, frozen yogurt, gelatin, pudding or custard, cottage cheese and fruit, juice, cold cereal, or a sandwich. These may be easier to take.

- Try salty or dry foods, such as bread or crackers. These may help calm your stomach.

- Rest between meals, but do not lie down completely flat. Elevate your upper body or sit up for at least two hours after eating.

- If the smell of food bothers you, ask someone else to cook; make sure the cooking area is well ventilated so that food smells don't linger.

- Avoid eating your favorite foods when you feel sick, so that you don't start to associate them with nausea and begin to dislike them.

- Drink a cup of herbal tea (chamomile or peppermint) with honey or a piece of fresh ginger, or chew on a small piece of fresh ginger root to help settle your stomach.

- If your medication seems to cause nausea, talk to your doctor or a pharmacist about timing your doses so that you take them when you are eating or right after you eat.

- Ask your doctor about taking anti-nausea medication. If one medication doesn't work, ask for a different one. Take the medication as directed— typically a half hour before meals.

Diarrhea is a problem for me.

Diarrhea can be caused by many things, including medications, stress, infections, or severe weight loss. Whatever the cause, diarrhea means that your body is not getting the fluids and nutrients it needs from the foods you eat. For this reason, it is critical that you pay attention to your fluid intake to prevent dehydration.

The following tips will help you deal with and lessen your diarrhea:

- Drink high-calorie fluids (at least eight glasses per day), such as juices, clear carbonated beverages, broth, and fruit or sports drinks. Water should not be the only fluid you drink, because it lacks the calories and nutrients your body must replace. Avoid drinks that have caffeine or alcohol; these stimulate the intestines and can cause further dehydration. Drink fluids at room temperature; very hot or cold fluids may stimulate the intestines and make diarrhea worse.

- Potassium is a vital mineral that is lost when you have diarrhea, and depletion can lead to muscle cramping and fatigue. Replace lost potassium by eating bananas, raisins, sports drinks, fruit juices (especially orange juice and nectars), vegetable juices, mashed potatoes, or canned fruits without seeds or skins.

- You may not feel like eating much, but skipping meals is not a good idea. Foods you may be able to tolerate are plain white rice, noodles, mashed potatoes, crackers, white toast, eggs, hot cereal, applesauce or other canned fruits without seeds or skins, bananas, gelatin, ice cream, sherbet, or broth-type soups.

- Avoid greasy or fatty foods that have large amounts of butter, margarine, or oils, and foods that are fried. For more tips, see the following discussion of fat intolerance.

- Avoid foods that are high in fiber or that have skins or seeds; these can be irritating and hard to digest. Avoid raw fruits and vegetables and whole-grain breads or cereals. Low-fiber foods, such as cooked vegetables, canned fruits without skins or seeds, ripe bananas, white rice, and white bread, are good choices.

- Avoid milk and milk products for a while. Drink low-fat milk and eat lean meats if you can tolerate them. Dairy aids containing lactase can help you digest and absorb the milk sugar that sometimes causes problems such as bloating and diarrhea (see the following discussion of lactose intolerance). Stick to plain boiled, baked, or broiled meats, and stay away from spicy foods or sauces.

- Cramps often accompany diarrhea and can be a sign of gas or air in your intestines. Carbonated beverages can worsen this problem and should be avoided. Foods that cause gas—such as raw apples, beans, cabbage, broccoli, cauliflower, onions, green peppers, and beer—should also be avoided.

- Ask your doctor about antidiarrheal medications. A tablespoon of Metamucil mixed with juice also may help control diarrhea, because the soluble fiber in it makes the stool bulky.

Note: If your diarrhea increases in frequency or lasts more than a week, consult your doctor. Unchecked diarrhea can cause further problems, such as dehydration and potassium loss, that must be prevented or corrected. Medications to help get diarrhea under control are available. (See Chapter 8, "Evaluating Common Symptoms of HIV/AIDS," for more information.)

What if I am constipated?

Constipation is often the result of not drinking enough fluids, not eating enough food or fiber, and not being physically active. Constipation may also develop as a side effect of certain medications, especially narcotic-based pain medications. In addition to drinking enough fluids, try these suggestions:

- Eat foods high in insoluble fiber, such as whole-grain breads and cereals, fresh fruits and vegetables, cooked beans and chickpeas, nuts, and seeds.

- Add small amounts of bran to food or liquids, to increase fiber.

- Include some aerobic exercise in your daily schedule.

- Ask your doctor about medications to relieve constipation.

I have trouble digesting fat (fat intolerance).

If you need to gain weight, fats are an excellent source of calories, but they can be hard to digest. Fat intolerance—difficulty digesting and absorbing fats—can be a problem for people with HIV/AIDS. If you experience discomfort after eating foods high in fat; you may need to reduce the amount of fat you eat. It is not usually a good idea to completely eliminate fat, unless you are having prolonged and severe diarrhea. If fat intolerance becomes a chronic problem, avoid all fat-rich foods, such as the ones listed in the accompanying table.

If your problem digesting fat is severe, products that contain no fat but have extra calories and protein are available. Other products have a special, easily digestible form of fat. These products may help you to keep your calorie intake and weight at appropriate levels.

Some people, particularly people who are taking HAART medications, may find they have lipodystrophy (fatty deposits on their bodies) and high blood cholesterol. These people won't need to try to digest fat—instead, they will need to avoid fats in the diet in order to lower blood cholesterol. If this sounds like you, you will want to eat fewer of the foods listed in "Foods High in Fat," below.

FOODS HIGH IN FAT		
• Fried foods	• Mayonnaise	• Whole milk
• Chips	• Pepperoni	• Luncheon meats
• Tuna in oil	• Cheeses	• Bacon
• French fries	• Cream sauces	• Gravies
• Salad dressing	• Hot dogs	• Peanut butter
• Chocolate	• Ice cream	• Doughnuts
• Rich desserts	• Sausages	
• Butter, oil, or margarine	• Cream or half-and-half	

I don't feel well when I eat dairy products (lactose intolerance).

If you notice that milk, cheese, and ice cream cause cramping, gas, bloating, or diarrhea, your body may be having trouble digesting lactose, a type of sugar found in milk and milk products. If your reactions subside with time, you can start eating these dairy foods again. After all, they are good protein sources.

The following suggestions can help you avoid the more troublesome dairy products and find ones you are able to tolerate:

- Avoid foods containing milk, such as pudding, custard, ice cream, cream soups, cream pies, gravies, and sauces. In place of milk, try nondairy products like enriched soy milk, rice milk, or other milk substitutes.

- Buy milk and milk products that contain an enzyme called *lactase,* which will help you digest lactose. Such items are found in the regular dairy section of your supermarket. Check the labels before buying.

- Some dairy products contain less lactose and therefore may be easier to tolerate. These include buttermilk, cottage cheese, sour cream, aged cheeses, sherbet, and yogurt.

- Look for kosher foods, labeled *pareve* or *parve* because they are milk-free.

- Take lactase pills or drops before eating food that has large amounts of lactose. You can buy these over the counter at any drugstore and at many grocery stores.

Dry mouth, mouth sores, and swallowing problems make it hard to eat anything.

Your mouth may feel dry as a side effect of some medications or from not drinking enough fluids. Also, infections in your mouth and throat can cause sores that make it painful to eat or swallow. The following tips may help you manage these symptoms:

- Avoid smoking and drinking alcohol; these irritate the mouth and throat.

- Soft foods that are smooth in consistency and easy to swallow are usually the easiest to eat. You can make swallowing easier by putting food through a blender, eating casseroles and stews, or adding butter, gravy, sauce, or salad dressing to moisten food. Choose dishes that don't have chunks of food in them. Add liquids to foods or dunk foods in soup, milk, juice, or hot chocolate. This makes them less irritating to your mouth and throat.

- Avoid spicy foods, foods with a high acid content (such as orange juice or tomatoes), and carbonated sodas. These can make mouth sores burn. Cold foods, such as ice pops, ice cream, sherbet, frozen yogurt, and thick milk shakes, can numb your mouth and are easy to swallow.

- If you find that you gag easily, avoid sticky foods, such as peanut butter, and slippery foods, such as gelatin.

- Use a straw for drinking fluids and a cup or glass for eating soup. Tilt your head back to make swallowing easier.

- Try eating soft, bland foods, such as pudding, custard, eggs, canned fruits, cottage cheese, yogurt, bananas, and creamed cereals.

- Avoid foods that require a lot of chewing or are tough and fibrous.

- Suck on sugar-free or sour hard candy, and on Popsicles or ice, or chew sugarless gum to stimulate salivation.

- Rinse your mouth frequently and drink lots of fluids to help with dryness. If dryness continues to be a problem even when you moisten your foods, your doctor or dentist may prescribe artificial saliva for you.

- Sleep with a humidifier in your room, and keep fluids by your bedside to sip on during the night if you are thirsty.

WHAT IF I HAVE OTHER HEALTH PROBLEMS?

Some people with HIV/AIDS who have developed diabetes or high cholesterol as a result of taking certain medications may need the following information to help control these conditions and prevent further complications.

Diabetes

If you have diabetes, it is important to watch the amount of carbohydrates you eat. Carbohydrates (starches and sugars) are the nutrients that break down into glucose. With the help of a hormone called *insulin,* the glucose is able to pass from the bloodstream into the body's cells, to be used as energy. When you have diabetes, however, either the body does not produce enough insulin or the cells cannot use the insulin produced. This means that glucose stays in the bloodstream and can cause complications. For this reason, limit the amount of foods you eat that are high in carbohydrates and eat equal-sized meals every four to five hours during the day.

The recommended amount of carbohydrates for each meal is forty-five to sixty grams, equal to about three to four servings of foods that are rich in carbohydrates, such as the starchy vegetables (potatoes, corn, beets, peas), breads, rice, pasta, and fruit. Each of these foods contains approximately fifteen grams of carbohydrate per portion. Most other vegetables are low in carbohydrates; these can usually be eaten in unlimited quantities because they contain only about five grams of carbohydrates per recommended serving. Other foods that should be limited include sweets (cakes, cookies, ice cream, etc.) and alcohol.

Although meat, fish, and poultry are low in carbohydrates, they do contain fat. Therefore, do not exceed the suggested portion size and number of servings per day (two to three ounces, three times per day). Refer to the Formula for Healthy Eating on page 236 and the Food Guide on pages 223–227 for more details.

People with diabetes have an increased risk of developing heart disease, circulatory problems, and high blood pressure. For this reason, it is important to reduce the fat, cholesterol, and sodium (salt) in the foods you eat, and to monitor your carbohydrate consumption. This, along with regular exercise, can help lower your blood sugar. It is also a good idea to take a class and learn more about managing diabetes.

High Cholesterol

If you have high cholesterol or high triglycerides (fats in the blood), it is a good idea to reduce the amount of fat and cholesterol you eat and to increase your fiber intake. Avoid the fatty foods listed in "Foods High in Fat"on page 248, and see "Hints for Reducing Fat in Your Eating Plan," below, and "Hints for Increasing Fiber in Your Eating Plan," page 253. These tips will help you to prevent the narrowing and hardening of the arteries that can cause heart attacks, and to control your blood pressure, blood sugar, and weight.

If you also have high blood pressure (hypertension), eat less salt and sodium. Read nutrition labels for sodium content, and experiment with herbs and spices to season your food. Unfortunately, many packaged, processed foods are high in sugar, fat, and sodium. If you eat these foods often, choose the brands that are lowest in sugar, fat, and sodium.

If you are dealing with diabetes or high cholesterol, be sure to consult a nutritionist to help determine the best eating plan for you. You may also need other medications to help control these problems.

HINTS FOR REDUCING FAT IN YOUR EATING PLAN

- Eat more poultry and fish, and less red meat (limit portions to 2–3 oz or 50–100 g—about the size of a deck of cards).

- Choose leaner cuts of meat.

- Trim the yellow fat and remove the skin from poultry.

- Eat egg yolks and organ meats (liver, kidneys, brains) in moderation.

- Broil, barbecue, or roast meats instead of frying them.

- Avoid deep-fried foods.

- Skim fat off stews and soups.

- Use low-fat or nonfat milk and milk products.

- Use fats (butter, margarine, oils, gravy, sauces, and salad dressings) sparingly (no more than 3–4 teaspoons or 15–20 ml per day).

- Use a nonstick pan with cooking oil spray.

HINTS FOR INCREASING FIBER IN YOUR EATING PLAN

- Build your meals around vegetables, grain products, and fruits.

- Eat a variety of fruits and vegetables, raw or lightly cooked.

- Eat low-fat grain products such as whole wheat breads, brown rice, and corn tortillas.

- Eat more lentils or beans and rice, and less meat.

- Snack on fruit or nonfat yogurt, not sweets or ice cream.

- Drink plenty of water to help move fiber through your system.

Changing your eating habits is not easy, and the suggestions provided in this chapter are only a start. The key to changing how you eat is to take an overall approach. This includes: making sure you're motivated, identifying what you're doing now, deciding what practical changes you can make and live with, and learning to solve any problems that come up. These steps really can be applied to all kinds of changes you want to make, and good self-managers use them all the time.

SUGGESTED READING

American Dietetic Association. *Living Well with HIV and AIDS: A Guide to Healthy Eating.* Chicago, Ill.: American Dietetic Association, 2003.

Duyff, Roberta L. *The American Dietetic Association's Complete Food and Nutrition Guide.* 2nd ed. Hoboken, N.J.: John Wiley & Sons, 2002.

American Heart Association. *Low-Fat, Low-Cholesterol Cookbook: Heart-Healthy, Easy-to-Make Recipes that Taste Great.* 2nd ed. New York: Clarkson Potter Publishers, 2001.

American Heart Association. *Low-Salt Cookbook: A Complete Guide to Reducing Sodium in Your Diet.* 2nd ed. New York: Clarkson Potter Publishers, 2002.

American Heart Association. *The New American Heart Association Cookbook.* 7th ed. New York: Clarkson Potter Publishers, 1998.

American Heart Association. *Quick & Easy Cookbook: More than 200 Healthful Recipes You Can Make in Minutes.* New York: Clarkson Potter Publishers, 1998.

Brody, Jane. *Jane Brody's Nutrition Book.* New York: Bantam Books, 1987.

Ferguson, James M., and Ferguson, Cassandra. *Habits Not Diets.* 4th ed. Boulder, Colo.: Bull Publishing, 2003.

Lappé, Frances. *Diet for a Small Planet.* New York: Ballantine, 1991.

Margen, Sheldon, and the editors of the U.C. Berkeley Wellness Letter. *Wellness Foods A to Z: An Indispensable Guide for Health-Conscious Food Lovers.* New York: Rebus Publishing, 2002.

Rinzler, Carol Ann. *The New Complete Book of Food: A Nutritional Medical and Culinary Guide.* New York: Checkmark Books, 1999.

Robertson, Laurel, Ruppenthal, Brian, and Flinders, Carol. *Laurel's Kitchen Caring: Recipes for Everyday Home Caregiving.* Berkeley, Calif.: Ten Speed Press, 1997.

Robertson, Laurel, Flinders, Carol, and Ruppenthal, Brian. *The New Laurel's Kitchen: A Handbook for Vegetarian Cookery and Nutrition.* Berkeley, Calif.: Ten Speed Press, 1986.

Web site for the American Dietetic Association. www.eatright.org. Accessed August 10, 2005.

Web site for the Federal Citizen Information Center. www.pueblo.gsa.gov. Accessed August 10, 2005.

CHAPTER THIRTEEN

Food Safety and Preparation Tips

J ust as you need to eat well when you have HIV disease, you must also protect yourself from bacteria that can cause food poisoning. People with HIV/AIDS are more likely than people with strong immune systems to acquire food-borne illnesses that can be hard to treat.

Food poisoning can cause nausea, vomiting, and diarrhea, all of which make you miserable and interfere with your eating. This, in turn, leads to weight loss, further weakens your immune system, and hastens the progression of the disease. Although for most people, food poisoning can be treated with rest and plenty of fluids, this is not true for people with HIV or AIDS. They may experience more serious and prolonged symptoms that are difficult to treat. They will require a doctor's care.

Because most food contamination results from the improper handling of food, you can protect yourself by following some basic safety guidelines when buying, preparing, serving, and storing foods. These guidelines are also important to keep in mind when eating away from home or traveling abroad.

FOOD HANDLING PRECAUTIONS

The American Dietetic Association recommends the following precautions for safety.

255

Shopping for Food

- Read food labels carefully. Avoid products that contain raw or under-cooked meat and dairy products. Avoid all dairy products that are not pasteurized.

- Check the dates on food packages. Don't buy or use packaged food whose "best if used by . . ." or expiration date has passed.

- Don't buy food with damaged packaging or food that has been handled or displayed improperly.

- Put packaged meat, poultry, or fish into a plastic bag before placing it in your shopping cart.

- When grocery shopping, select cold and frozen foods last, and ask that these foods be packed in the same bag.

- Carry a cooler in your car to store the cold and frozen foods if the trip home takes longer than thirty minutes.

- Check your refrigerator regularly and throw away foods whose expiration date has passed.

Food Storage

- Storing foods properly is the key to food safety. Be sure to refrigerate or freeze foods that require cold storage as soon as possible after buying them. The temperature in your refrigerator should be 40°F or lower, and the freezer temperature should be 0°F or lower. Use a refrigerator thermometer to make sure temperatures are in the proper range. See "Lifespan of Refrigerated Products," page 258.

- Label your stored foods with the date of purchase, and follow the recommended storage times for each type of food. Foods that contain harmful bacteria do not always look or smell spoiled. When in doubt, throw it out.

- Always thaw frozen foods in the refrigerator or microwave. Do not allow drippings from defrosting foods (especially meat, poultry, or fish) to touch other foods in the refrigerator. Place them in a separate container on the bottom shelf of the refrigerator to thaw.

- Put leftover prepared foods containing meat, eggs, or milk products in the refrigerator or freezer immediately. Store the portions in small containers for easy use later.

- Cover food tightly with plastic wrap or store in airtight containers.

- Don't eat leftovers that have been in the refrigerator for more than two days.

Food Preparation and Cooking

- Always begin by washing your hands with soapy water. Remember to wash your hands again after handling any raw foods and before handling cooked food.

- Don't use wooden cutting boards for meat, poultry, or fish. Instead, use plastic boards, which are easier to sanitize, or disposable cutting sheets.

- Clean all utensils, plastic cutting boards, and chipped china or crockery in the dishwasher, or wash them in hot, soapy water (at least 140°F) and rinse them well.

- Sanitize your plastic cutting board after working with raw meats, fish, and poultry. Soak the board for ten minutes in a solution of one to two tablespoons of bleach per gallon of warm water.

- Clean utensils, countertops, shelves, refrigerator, and freezer with the bleach-and-warm water solution as an additional safety step.

- Keep towels and sponges clean. Replace sponges often, and use different sponges for washing dishes and for other types of cleaning. Put wet sponges in microwave oven and heat for two minutes.

Meat, poultry, and fish

- Never eat raw meat, poultry, or fish of any kind. Even steak tartare, carpaccio, raw oysters, raw shrimp, sashimi, or sushi topped with raw fish can cause serious infections.

LIFESPAN OF REFRIGERATED PRODUCTS STORED AT 35° TO 40°F	
Food Product	**Use Within**
• Raw beefsteak and roasts, raw pork chops, raw lamb chops and roasts, cooked ham, lunch meat	3–5 days
• Ground beef, turkey, pork, or lamb; sausage	1–2 days
• Hot dogs	1 week
• Raw chicken or turkey, giblets, fish	1–2 days
• Leftover cooked meat and meat dishes; soups and stews	3–4 days
• Leftover gravy and meat broth	1–2 days
• Leftover cooked poultry and poultry dishes	3–4 days
• Leftover cooked poultry covered with broth or gravy; leftover chicken nuggets, patties, or fried chicken	1–2 days
• Fresh eggs in the shell	3 weeks
• Raw egg yolks or whites (out of the shell)	2–4 days
• Hard-cooked eggs	1 week

- Cook all meats to 165°F or higher. Cook poultry to 180°F. Use a meat thermometer to check the temperature.

- Cook all meats completely. Red meat should be well-done, and poultry should be cooked until the juices are clear.

- Reheat all leftovers thoroughly, to 165°F or higher.

- When barbecuing, precook meats just before putting them on the grill to make sure that the inside reaches the proper temperature.

- Eat meats and meat dishes while they are hot, and store leftovers in the refrigerator immediately. Don't let them sit out at room temperature for more than two hours.

Eggs

- Check at the store to make sure you don't buy eggs with cracked shells. Refrigerate eggs as soon as you get home. Never let eggs or dishes prepared with eggs sit out at room temperature.

- Don't eat raw eggs or eggs that are soft-boiled, or scrambled but runny. Avoid foods prepared with uncooked or undercooked eggs, such as Caesar salad dressing, chocolate mousse, some frostings, homemade eggnog, and homemade mayonnaise. If you eat homemade ice cream, check to see whether raw eggs are an ingredient.

- When cooking eggs, make sure the yolk and white are firm. Follow these cooking times and temperatures:

  - Scrambled eggs: Cook for one minute at medium setting (250°F for electric frying pans).

  - Sunny-side up eggs: Cook for seven minutes at medium setting (250°F), or cook covered for four minutes at 250°F.

  - Fried, over-easy eggs: Cook for three minutes at medium setting on one side, then for one minute on the other side.

  - Poached eggs: Cook for five minutes in boiling water.

  - Hard-boiled eggs: Cook for at least seven minutes in boiling water.

- Use a pasteurized, frozen egg product—not raw eggs—in recipes for uncooked dishes.

Milk and dairy products

- Buy only pasteurized milk and dairy products. Read the labels on cheeses, as not all of them are pasteurized.

- Check the expiration date. Buy products before the expiration date, and use within the next several days.

- Don't eat soft-ripened cheeses or cheese that has mold on it. Throw away moldy cheese.

Fruits and vegetables

- Choose fresh fruits and vegetables with unbroken skins.

- Wash all fruits and vegetables thoroughly and peel those with skin.

- Avoid fruits and vegetables that are moldy or have soft spots that show signs of rotting or mold.

- Refrigerate to reduce spoilage.

Eating Out

- Be sure your eating utensils, place settings, and beverage glasses are clean. Don't be shy about returning dirty utensils or food that is not hot enough or not cooked thoroughly.

- In a restaurant, avoid eating the same foods that you avoid eating at home.

- Avoid salad bars. You can't be sure how well the vegetables or fruits have been washed or handled, or how long they have been sitting out. If you are given a choice between salad and soup, choose the soup.

- Order meats medium-well to well-done. To check doneness, cut into the center of the meat. If it is pink or bloody, it needs to be cooked more. Fish should be flaky, not rubbery, when cut.

- Order eggs cooked on both sides, and don't eat runny-looking eggs.

- If you are not sure about the ingredients and preparation of a dish, ask before ordering.

- Don't eat raw or even lightly-steamed seafood.

Traveling Abroad

- Boil all water before drinking.

- Drink only beverages made with boiled water, and canned or bottled carbonated drinks. Use only ice cubes that have been made from boiled water.

- Avoid uncooked vegetables and salads.

- Peel all fruit.

- Eat cooked foods while they are still hot.

SAFETY AND ENJOYMENT

After reading these chapters, you may feel that we have taken all the fun out of food and made eating a big hassle. Luckily, however, it doesn't have to be that way. Although you may need to modify what you eat and follow some basic food safety guidelines, these changes are not always difficult to make. In fact, everyone should practice these same safety measures. With a little thought, planning, and practice, mealtime can be one of the best parts of your day. By making healthy choices and taking safety precautions, you will enjoy your food more and feel more in control of your health!

PART FIVE

Managing Personal and Practical Issues

CHAPTER FOURTEEN

Communicating

You just don't understand! How often has this statement, expressed or unexpressed, summed up a frustrating verbal exchange? The first goal in any communication between you and someone else is that the other person understand what you are trying to say. Feeling that you are not understood leads to frustration, and a prolonged feeling of frustration can lead to depression, anger, and helplessness. These are not good feelings for anyone, especially people with chronic illness. Dealing with HIV/AIDS can be frustrating enough without adding communication problems.

Poor communication is the biggest factor in poor relationships, whether between spouses, family members and friends, coworkers, or doctors and patients. (For a more detailed discussion on communication with your doctor, see Chapter 4, "Working with Your Doctor.") Even in casual relationships, poor communication causes frustration. For example, think how often you have been angry and frustrated as a customer, and how often this is because of poor communication?

When you have a chronic illness, good communication becomes a necessity. As a self-manager, it is in your best interest to learn the skills necessary to make the communications in your life as effective as possible. In this chapter, we discuss ways to improve the communication process: How to express feelings in a positive way, how to ask for help, how to say "no," how to listen, and how to get more information from the other person.

While reading this chapter, keep in mind that *communication is a two-way street*. As uncomfortable as you may feel about expressing your feelings and asking for help, chances are that others are also feeling this way. It may be up to you to make sure the lines of communication are open.

VERBALIZING FEELINGS: "I" MESSAGES

Let's face it, many of us are uncomfortable expressing our feelings, especially if doing so means we may seem critical of the person to whom we're talking. Yet when emotions are high, attempts to express frustration can be laden with "you" messages. *You* can be an accusatory word, suggesting blame. Its use, when expressing feelings, can cause the other person to feel as though he or she is under attack. Suddenly, the other person feels on the defensive, and protective barriers go up. The person trying to express feelings, in turn, feels greater anxiety, and the situation escalates to anger, frustration, and bad feelings.

I, on the other hand, is not an accusatory word. It doesn't strike out or blame. When expressing your own feelings, express them in terms of how *you* feel, not how the other person *makes you* feel.

Following are some examples of "you" and "I" messages.

"You" Message Example

Partner 1:   You never seem to be interested in sex anymore. I wish you would just try to show some interest.

Partner 2:   You seem to have nothing on your mind except sex. I just have so many other things to worry about right now . . . juggling my meds, exercising, eating right.

Partner 1:   But what about my needs? Why don't you make that one of your priorities? You're being very self-centered.

Partner 2:   ME self-centered? All you think about is sex, and you're calling me self-centered!?!

Partner 1:   Well, I can see once again that talking about this is getting us nowhere. It just makes it all worse!

"I" Message Example

Partner 1:   I really miss having sex with you. It's been awhile, hasn't it?

Partner 2:   Yes, it has. I just feel so overwhelmed with trying to adjust to the medication schedules and doctor appointments, and trying to focus on staying healthy, that I don't have as much energy as I used to.

Partner 1:   I never really thought about how much more complicated your life has become with all the new pills you're taking. Still, I miss feeling close and intimate. Having sex always helped me feel closer to you.

Partner 2:   I really miss that, too, but I just don't have the energy for having sex. I feel tired most of the time.

Partner 1:   Maybe if we just spend some time alone holding each other and talking, that will help me feel close to you again.

Partner 2:   That would really feel great. I miss cuddling with you at night, but I didn't want to make you think I was initiating sex. If we can just hold each other, that would be a big load off my mind.

Partner 1:   That sounds like a great compromise to me. And maybe we can come up with some ideas on how I can help you with the details in your life.

The trick to "I" messages is to avoid the use of the word *you* and instead express your personal feelings using the word *I*. Of course, like any new skill, "I" messages take practice. Start by really listening, to both yourself and to others. Take some of the "you" messages you hear and turn them into "I" messages in your head. By playing this little word game in your head, you'll be surprised at how fast "I" messages become a habit in your own expressions.

There are some things to keep in mind when using "I" messages. First, they are not a miracle cure. Sometimes the listener has to have time to hear them. This is especially true if "you" messages and blaming have been the more usual ways of communicating. Even if at first using "I" messages seems ineffective, continue to use them and refine your skill. Some people may use "I" messages as a means of manipulation. If used in this way, problems can escalate. To be used effectively, "I" messages must report honest feelings.

Note: "I" messages are an excellent way to express positive feelings and compliments! "I really appreciate the extra time you gave me today."

ASKING FOR HELP

Problems communicating about the subject of help are pretty common. For some reason, people feel awkward asking for help or refusing help. Although this problem is universal, it can come up more often for people with HIV/AIDS.

It may be emotionally difficult for some of us to ask for needed help. Maybe it's difficult for us to admit to ourselves that we are unable to do things as easily as we could in the past. When this is the case, try to avoid hedging your request with: "I'm sorry to have to ask this . . ."; "I know this is asking a lot . . ."; or "I hate to ask this, but . . . ." Hedging tends to put the other person on the defensive ("Gosh, what's he going to ask for that's

"I" MESSAGE EXERCISE

Change the following statements into "I" messages. (Watch out for hidden "you" messages!) When you finish the exercise, compare your "I" messages with our suggestions.

1. You expect me to wait on you hand and foot!

2. You hardly ever touch me anymore. You don't pay any attention to me since I tested positive.

3. You don't tell me the side effects of all these drugs you're giving me or why I have to take them, doctor.

Sample answers to "I" Message Exercise:

1. I'm frustrated by your illness. I feel as though I'm doing more than my share right now.

2. I'm concerned that we seem to have grown apart since I tested positive.

3. I don't feel well informed about the drugs I'm taking, doctor. *Or:* I feel I need to understand more about the medications I'm taking.

such a big deal, anyway?"). Be specific about what help you are requesting. A general request can lead to misunderstanding, and the other person can react negatively to insufficient information.

General request: "I know this is the last thing you want to do, but I need help moving. Will you help me?'

Reaction: "Uh . . . well . . . I don't know. Um . . . can I get back to you after I check my schedule?" (Probably next year!)

Specific request: "I'm moving next week, and I'd like to move my books and kitchen stuff ahead of time. Would you mind helping me load and unload the boxes in my car Saturday morning? I think it can be done in one trip."

Reaction: "I'm busy Saturday morning, but I could give you a hand Friday night, if you'd like."

People with chronic illness must also sometimes deal with offers of help that are not needed or desired. In most cases, these offers come from people who are dear to you and genuinely want to be helpful. A well-worded "I" message can refuse the help tactfully, without embarrassing the other person: "Thank you for being so thoughtful, but today I think I can handle it myself. I'd like to be able to take you up on your offer another time though!"

RESPONDING TO OTHERS' REQUESTS

Suppose you are the one being asked to help someone. Often we need more information before we can respond to a request. Without enough information we often tend to say no. The example we just discussed about helping a person move is a good one. "Help me move" can mean anything from "Help me move furniture upstairs" to "Please pick up the pizza for the hungry troops." It is important to understand what the *specific* request is before responding. *Asking for more information* or *paraphrasing* the request will often help clarify it. It's a good idea to begin with a phrase such as "Before I answer. . . ." Hopefully, this will prevent the person whom you are paraphrasing from feeling sure that you are going to say yes.

Once you know what the specific request is, if you decide to decline, it is important to *acknowledge the importance of the request* to the other person. In this way, the person will see that you are rejecting the *request*, rather than the *person*. Your turn-down should not be a put-down. "You know, that's a worthwhile project you're doing, but I think it's beyond my capabilities this week." Again, specifics are the key. Try to be clear about the conditions of your turn-down. Will you always turn down this request, or is it just today or this week or right now that it's a problem?

LISTENING

Listening is probably the most important communication skill. Most of us are much better at talking than we are at listening. You need to actually listen to what the other person is *saying and feeling*. Unfortunately, most of us are often already preparing a response instead of just listening while the other person is speaking.

There are several levels involved in being a good listener:

1. *Listen to the words and tone of voice, and observe body language.* Sometimes it is difficult to begin a conversation if there is a problem. There may be times when words alone don't tell you there is something bothering this person. Is the voice wavering? Does he or she appear to be struggling to find "the right words"? Do you notice body tension? Does he or she seem distracted? If you pick up on some of these signs, this person probably has more on his or her mind than words are expressing.

2. *Acknowledge having heard the other person.* Let the person know you heard him or her. This may be a simple "uh huh." Many times the only thing the other person wants is acknowledgment, or just someone to listen. Sometimes merely talking to a sympathetic listener is helpful.

3. *Acknowledge the content of the problem.* Let the other person know you understood the content and emotional level of the problem. You can do this by restating what you heard—for example, the content: "You are planning a trip." Or you can respond by acknowledging the emotions: "That must be difficult" or "You seem sad about it." When you respond on an emotional level, the results are often startling. These responses tend to open the gates for more expression of feelings and thoughts. Responding to either the content or emotion can also help communication by discouraging the other person from repeating himself or herself.

4. *Respond by seeking more information.* This is especially important if you are not completely clear about what is being said or what is wanted. There is more than one useful method for seeking and getting information.

GETTING MORE INFORMATION

Getting more information from another person is a bit of an art. Some of these methods are simple; others are more subtle.

Ask for More

Asking is the simplest way to get more information. "Tell me more" will probably get you more, as will "I don't understand . . . please explain"; "I'd like to know more about. . . "; "Could you put that another way?"; "How do you mean?"; "I'm not sure I got that"; and "Could you expand on that?"

Paraphrase

Paraphrasing is a good tool if you want to make sure you understand what the other person meant (not just what he or she *said*). Paraphrasing can either help or hinder effective communication, though, depending on the way the paraphrase is worded. It is important to remember to paraphrase in the form of a *question*, not a statement:

Original statement:	"Well, I don't know. I'm really not feeling up to par. This party will be crowded, there'll probably be smokers there, and I really don't know the hosts very well, anyway."
Paraphrased as a statement:	"Obviously, you're telling me you don't want to go to the party."

| *Paraphrased as a question:* | "Are you saying that you'd rather stay home than go to the party?" |

The response to the first paraphrase may be anger: "No, I didn't say that! If you're going to be that way, I'll stay home for sure." Or the response may be no response at all—a total shutdown of communication, resulting from either anger or despair ("He just doesn't understand"). People don't like to be told what they meant.

The response to the second paraphrase may be more open: "That's not what I meant. I'm just feeling a little nervous about meeting new people. I'd really like it if you'd stay near me during the party. I'd feel better about it and I might have a good time."

As you see, the second paraphrase promotes further communication, and an explanation of the real reason the person was expressing doubt about the party. You get more information from the second paraphrase (the question) and no new information from the first one (the statement).

Be Specific

If you want specific information, you must ask specific questions. We often speak in generalities:

| *Doctor:* | How have you been feeling? |

| *Patient:* | Not so good. |

The doctor's question doesn't produce much in the way of information about the patient's condition. "Not so good" isn't very useful. Here's how the doctor gets more information:

| *Doctor:* | Are you still having those sharp pains in your left arm? |

| *Patient:* | Yes. A lot. |

| *Doctor:* | How often? |

Patient: A couple of times a day.

Doctor: How long do they last?

Patient: A long time.

Doctor: About how many minutes, would you say?

And so on. Physicians have been trained to get specific information from patients, but most of us have not been trained to ask specific questions. Again, simply *asking for specifics* often works: "Can you be more specific about . . . ?"; "Are you thinking of something particular?" If you want to know "why," be specific about what it is. If you ask a specific question, you will be more likely to get a specific answer.

Simply asking "Why?" can unnecessarily prolong your attempt to get specific information. In addition to being a general, rather than a specific, word, *why* makes a person think in terms of cause and effect, and he or she may respond at a level entirely different from what you had in mind. Most of us have witnessed a three-year-old who keeps asking "Why?" over and over again until the information he or she wants is finally obtained (or the parent runs from the room, screaming). The poor parent doesn't have the faintest idea what the child has in mind, and repeatedly answers, "Because . . ." in increasingly specific order until the child's question is answered. Sometimes, however, the direction the answers take is entirely different from the subject of the child's question, and the child never gets the information he or she wanted. Rather than *why*, begin your questions with *who, which, when, where,* or *what.* These words promote a specific response. For example:

Doctor: I'm going to send you for a colonoscopy.

Patient: Why?

Doctor.   Well, because I feel that anyone with blood in his stool should have one.

WORDS THAT CAN HELP OR HINDER	
Words that Help	**Words that Hinder**
• I	• You
• Right now, at this time, at this point, today	• Never, always, every time, constantly
• Who, which, where, when	• Obviously . . .
• How do you mean? Please explain.	• Why?
• Tell me more. I don't understand.	

Patient: Why is that?

Doctor: It's medically indicated.

And so on. This questioning could go on for a long time, while the patient's "Why?" question may hide any number of different concerns. Compare the conversation above with this one:

Doctor: I'm going to send you for a colonoscopy.

Patient: What do you think might be wrong?

Doctor: I'm not sure. It's probably not serious, but you could have colon cancer.

Patient: Who does the colonoscopy? You?

Doctor: No, Dr. Jones, the GI specialist, will do it.

And so on. Asking specific questions like these helps you communicate better and helps prevent misunderstandings.

Good communication skills help make life easier for everyone, especially when HIV/AIDS enters the picture. The skills discussed in this chapter should help smooth the communication process and bring you closer to your loved ones.

SUGGESTED READING

Beck, Aaron T. *Love Is Never Enough: How Couples Can Overcome Misunderstandings, Resolve Conflicts, and Solve Relationship Problems Through Cognitive Therapy.* New York: Harper and Row, 1988.

Burley-Allen, Madelyn. *Listening: The Forgotten Skill: A Self-Teaching Guide.* 2nd ed. New York: John Wiley & Sons, 1995.

Jones, J. Alfred, Kreps, Gary L., and Phillips, Gerald M. *Communicating with Your Doctor: Getting the Most out of Health Care.* Cresskill, N.J.: Hampton Press, 1995.

McKay, Matthew, Fanning, Patrick, and Paleg, Kim. *Couple Skills: Making Your Relationship Work.* Oakland, Calif.: New Harbinger Publications, 1994.

McKay, Matthew, Davis, Martha, and Fanning, Patrick. *Messages: The Communication Skills Book.* 2nd ed. Oakland, Calif.: New Harbinger Publications, 1995.

CHAPTER FIFTEEN

Making Your Wishes Known: Advance Directives

A ll of us, whether ill or healthy, have feelings about our own death. Death may be feared, welcomed, accepted, or—all too often— pushed aside to be thought about at some other time. Somewhere, in the back of our minds, though, most of us have ideas about how and when we would like to die. For some of us, life is so important that we feel that everything should be done to sustain it. For others, life is important only so long as we can be active participants. For many people, the issue isn't really death but, rather, dying. We may have heard about the eighty-year-old who died skiing. This may be considered a "good death." On the other hand, we may have a friend who died after spending a long time in a nursing home, unaware of his or her surroundings. This is usually not what we would wish for ourselves.

Although none of us can have absolute control over our own death, it is something that, like the rest of life, we can help manage. That is, we can express our wishes, make decisions, and probably add a great deal to the quality of our death. Proper management can lessen the negative impact of death on our survivors.

This chapter presents information that will help you better manage some of the legal issues of death, using legal documents called *advance directives*. As you read this chapter, bear in mind that each state has different laws about advance directives. You can get information and forms specific for your state by contacting the National Hospice and Palliative Care

Organization. They can be reached at 1-800-989-WILL (9455) or online at the Caring Connections Web site at www.caringinfo.org.

LIVING WILL

The living will is probably the best known of the advance directives. It allows you to legally refuse life-support measures when you are considered to be near the end of your life—usually within six months.

The living will is widely available and serves a useful purpose. However, it is much less flexible than other advance directives, such as the durable power of attorney for health care (DPAHC). Remember, too, that the living will does not have legal standing in every state. Be sure to find out what your options are.

DURABLE POWER OF ATTORNEY FOR HEALTH CARE

A durable power of attorney for health care (DPAHC) lets you do two things: (1) state your wishes about the kind of medical care you would like to receive; and (2) appoint an *agent* to make health care decisions for you when you cannot do so for yourself. A DPAHC, like a living will, can help protect you from "heroic" lifesaving measures if you do not want them. However, the two documents have some important differences.

- A living will is good only in case of a terminal illness, whereas a DPAHC can apply to any illness.

- A living will enables you only to refuse treatment, whereas a DPAHC allows you to accept, refuse, or withdraw different forms of treatment.

- A living will does not allow you to appoint an agent. A DPAHC does.

In your DPAHC, you can include guidelines for your agent about what kind of health care you would like, under what circumstances. For example, you may indicate that you want everything possible done to keep you alive, no matter what your condition; or you may ask that you not receive any treatment or food if you are in a coma or near death. Although you do not have to write down your wishes, doing so can be reassuring for family members and for doctors who see your DPAHC form.

Note that it is especially important to have a durable power of attorney for health care if you wish to choose your partner or someone who is not a blood relative as your agent. Otherwise, it's possible that your medical decisions will end up being made by a family member who may be unaware of or disagree with your wishes.

The agent named in your durable power of attorney for health care has the power to make medical decisions for you only when you are unable to make decisions yourself (for example, if you are in a coma or are taking medications that affect your alertness). The agent can make decisions only about your medical care, not about finances or other matters.

The durable power of attorney offers great flexibility and can be more useful than a living will. However, it may not be legally recognized in your state. Be sure to check. Some states have advance directives in addition to the living will and DPAHC, which we do not cover here.

Creating a DPAHC means making many decisions. In the following section we cover each of the major issues likely to appear on your state's DPAHC form.

Choosing a Health Care Agent

Begin by deciding who you want as your agent. The person can be a friend or family member, but cannot be the physician who is providing your care. There are some considerations to be made in choosing your agent. First, the person should generally be available in the geographic area where you live. If the agent is not available to make decisions for you, he or she is not much help. Just to be on the safe side, you can also name a backup agent, who would act in your behalf if your first-choice agent were not available. Second, you must be sure that this person thinks like you think or at least is willing to carry out your wishes. Third, the person must be someone who you feel would be able to carry out your wishes. Sometimes a partner or child is not the best agent because this person is too close to you emotionally. For example, if you wish not to be resuscitated while in a severe coma, your agent has to be able to tell the doctor not to resuscitate. This decision could be difficult or impossible for a family member or partner to make on the spot. Be sure the person you choose as your agent is up to such a task. Finally, you want your agent to be someone who will not find this job too much of an emotional burden. Thus, the person has to be comfortable with the role, and willing and able to carry out your wishes.

In review, look for these characteristics in an agent:

- Someone who is likely to be available should he or she need to act on your behalf

- Someone who understands your wishes and is willing to carry them out

- Someone who is emotionally prepared and able to carry out your wishes

- Someone who will not be emotionally burdened by carrying out your wishes

As you see, finding the right agent is a very important task. You may want to talk to several people before making your choice; these may be the most important interviews you ever conduct. We talk more about discussing your wishes with family, friends, and your doctor later in this chapter.

Your Wishes Concerning Medical Treatment

The other major decision you'll need to make has to do with the kind of medical care you would like, under what circumstances. In other words, what are your directions to your agent? Some DPAHC forms give you several statements to choose from, or leave a space in which you can write your own statement. Here are some sample statements:

I do *not* want my life to be prolonged and I do *not* want life-sustaining treatment to be provided or continued if: (1) I am in an irreversible coma or persistent vegetative state; (2) I am terminally ill and the application of life-sustaining procedures would serve only to artificially delay the moment of my death; or (3) under any other circumstances where the burdens of treatment outweigh the expected benefits. I want my agent to consider the relief of suffering and the quality and extent or possible extension of my life in making decisions concerning life-sustaining treatment.

I want my life to be prolonged and I want life-sustaining treatment to be provided *unless I am in a coma or vegetative state* that my doctor reasonably believes to be irreversible. Once my doctor has reasonably concluded that I will remain unconscious for the rest of my life, I do *not* want life-sustaining treatment to be provided or continued.

I want my life to be prolonged to the greatest extent possible without regard to my condition, my chances for recovery, or the cost of the procedures.

Some DPAHC forms simply make a "general statement of authority granted," in which you give your agent full power to make decisions. You do not write out the details of these decisions; you simply trust your agent to follow your wishes. Because these wishes are not explicitly written, it is very important that you discuss them in detail with your agent.

Other Statements of Desires, Special Provisions, or Limitations

All DPAHC forms also have a space in which you can write out specific wishes that either limit or add to the authority you have given your agent. You are not required to give specific details but may wish to. Knowing what details to write is a little complicated because you do not know the exact circumstances in which the agent will have to act. However, you can get some idea by asking your doctor about what he or she thinks are the things most likely to happen to someone with your condition. Then you can direct your agent how to act. Your specific directions can cover outcomes, specific circumstances, or both. If you discuss outcomes, the statement should focus on which types of outcomes would be acceptable and which would not—for example, "Resuscitate if I can continue to fully function mentally."

Following are two of the common circumstances encountered by people with HIV/AIDS.

- *AIDS dementia complex* is a disease that can leave you with little or no mental function. In spite of this, it is generally not life-threatening, at least not for a long time. However, people with AIDS dementia complex may be vulnerable to other ailments that can become life threatening—such as pneumonia, meningitis, and wasting. What you need to decide is how much treatment you would want if you were to have AIDS dementia complex. For example, would you want antibiotics if you got pneumonia? Would you want to be resuscitated if you died in your sleep? Would you like a feeding tube if you become unable to feed yourself? Remember, it is your choice how to answer each of these questions. You may not want to be resuscitated, but you may want a feeding tube. You may want to use all means to sustain life or, more conservatively, you may not want any special means used to sustain life.

- You may have *very poor lung function* that will not improve. Should you be unable to breathe on your own, would you want to be placed in an intensive care unit on mechanical ventilation (a breathing machine)? Remember, this is a situation in which you will not improve. To say that you never want ventilation is very different from saying that you don't want it if it is used to sustain life when no improvement is likely. Obviously, mechanical ventilation can be lifesaving in crises such as a severe asthma attack, when it is used for a short time while the body regains normal function. Here the issue is not whether to use mechanical ventilation *ever*, but rather, when—under what circumstances—you wish it to be used.

These examples should give you some idea of the directions to give in your durable power of attorney for health care. Again, to better understand how to write such directions and how to personalize them to your own condition, you may want to talk with your physician about the most common problems and decision making for people like you.

In summary, there are several decisions you need to make in directing your agent on how to act on your behalf:

- Generally, *how much treatment do you want?* This can range from the very aggressive—that is, doing many things to sustain life—to the very conservative—doing almost nothing to sustain life, except to keep you clean and comfortable.

- Given the types of life-threatening things likely to happen to people with your condition, *what sorts of treatment do you want and under what conditions?*

- If you become *mentally incapacitated*, what sorts of treatment do you want for *other illnesses*, such as pneumonia?

Many people get this far. That is, they have thought through their wishes about dying and have even written them down in a DPAHC. This is an excellent beginning, but not the end of the job. A good manager has to do more than just write a memo. He or she has to see that the memo gets delivered. If you really want your wishes carried out, you must share them fully with your agent, your family, and your doctor. This is often not an easy task. In the following pages, we discuss ways to make these conversations easier.

TALKING WITH YOUR FAMILY, FRIENDS, AND AGENT

Before you can discuss your wishes with family, friends, and agent, all interested parties need to have copies of your DPAHC. Once you have completed the documents, have them witnessed and signed. In some states they may also need to be notarized. Make several copies at any copy center. You will need copies for your agent, family members, and your doctor. You may also want to give one to your lawyer.

Now you are ready to talk about your wishes. Nobody likes to discuss his or her own death, or that of a loved one. Therefore, it is not surprising that when you bring up this subject the response is often, "Oh, don't think about that," or "That's a long time off," or "Don't be so morbid, you're not that sick." Unfortunately, this is usually enough to end the conversation. Your job as a self-manager is to keep the conversation open. Here are some suggestions to begin your discussion of this subject:

- *Prepare your durable power of attorney*, and then give copies to the appropriate friends or family members. *Ask them to read it* and then set a specific time to discuss it. If they give you one of those responses mentioned on page 285, say that you understand this is a difficult topic, but it is important to you to discuss it with them. This is a good time to practice the "I" messages discussed in Chapter 14, "Communicating." For example, "I understand that death is a difficult thing to talk about. However, it is very important to me that we have this discussion."

- Get *blank copies* of the DPAHC form for those who are close to you and suggest that *you each fill one out and share them with each other*. Present this task as an important aspect of being a mature adult or family member. Making this a group project involving everyone may make it easier to discuss. Besides, it will help to clarify everyone's values about the topics of death and dying.

- If these two suggestions seem too difficult or are for some reason impossible to carry out, *write a letter* or prepare an *audiotape* to send to the people closest to you or members of your family. In the letter or tape, say why you feel your death is an important topic to discuss and that you want them to know your wishes. Then state your wishes, providing reasons for your choices. At the same time, send each person a copy of your DPAHC. Ask that they each respond in some way, or set aside some time to talk in person or on the phone.

TALKING WITH YOUR DOCTOR

From our research we have learned that, in general, people have a much more difficult time talking to their doctors about their wishes surrounding death than to their families. In fact, only a very small percentage of people who have written DPAHCs ever share these with their physicians. There are several reasons why it is important that such a discussion take place. First, you need to *be sure that your doctor has values that are compatible with your wishes.* If you and your doctor do not have the same values, it may be difficult for him or her to carry out your wishes. Second, *your doctor needs to know what you want.* This allows him or her to take appropriate actions, such as writing orders to resuscitate or not to use mechanical resuscitation should this be needed. Third, *your doctor needs to know who your agent is and how to contact this person.* If an important decision has to be made and your wishes are to be followed, the doctor must talk with your agent. It is important to give your doctor a copy of your durable power of attorney for health care, so that it can become a permanent part of your medical record.

As surprising as it may seem, many physicians also find it difficult to discuss death and how it may occur with their patients. After all, they are in the business of helping to keep people alive and well. They don't like to think about their patients dying. On the other hand, most doctors want their patients to have durable powers of attorney for health care. This relieves them of pressure and worry.

If you wish, *plan a time with your doctor when you can discuss your wishes.* This should not be a side conversation at the end of a regular visit. Rather, start a visit by saying, "I want a few minutes to discuss with you my wishes in the event of a serious problem or impending death." When you put it this way, most doctors will make time to talk with you. If the doctor says that he or she does not have enough time, then ask when you can make another appointment to talk about it. This is a situation in which you may need to be a little assertive. Sometimes a doctor, like your family members or friends, may say, "Oh, you don't have to worry about that, let me do it," or "We'll worry about that when the time comes." Again, you will have to take the initiative, using an "I" message to communicate that this is important to you and that you do not want to put off the discussion.

Sometimes doctors do not want to worry you. They think they are doing you a favor by not describing all the unpleasant things that may happen to you, or the potential treatments, in the case of serious problems. You can help your doctor by telling him or her that having control and making some decisions about your future will ease your mind. Not knowing or not being clear on what will happen is more worrisome than being faced with the facts, unpleasant as they may be, and dealing with them.

Even if you are aware of all of the above, it is still sometimes hard to talk with your doctor. Therefore, it may also be helpful to *bring your agent with you* when you have this discussion. The agent can facilitate the discussion and, at the same time, meet your doctor. This way, everyone has a chance to clarify any misunderstandings about your wishes. It opens the lines of communication so that if your agent and physician have to act to carry out your wishes, they can do so with few problems.

So now you have done all the important things. You can rest easy. The hard work is over. However, remember that you can change your mind at any time. Your agent may no longer be available, or your wishes may change. Be sure to keep your durable power of attorney for health care updated. Like any legal document, it can be revoked or changed at any time.

Making your wishes known about how you want to be treated in case of serious or life-threatening illness is one of the most important tasks of self-management. The best way to do this is to prepare a DPAHC and share it with your family, close friends, and physician.

AN IMPORTANT RESOURCE

CARING CONNECTIONS

Toll-free Help Line: (800) 658-8898

E-mail: caringinfo@nhpco.org

Web site: www.caringinfo.org

Street Address:
National Hospice and Palliative Care Organization

1700 Diagonal Road, Suite 625

Alexandria, Virginia 22314

Telephone: (703) 837-1500

Fax: (703) 837-1233

Be sure to check on your state's appropriate forms by asking your doctor or lawyer or by writing to Caring Connections. You can also get the forms from the Caring Connections Web site (see "An Important Resource," page 286, for contact information).

SUGGESTED READING

Cantor, Norman L. *Advance Directives and the Pursuit of Death with Dignity.* Bloomington, Ind.: Indiana University Press, 1993.

King, Nancy M. P. *Making Sense of Advance Directives.* Washington, D.C.: Georgetown University Press, 1996.

CHAPTER SIXTEEN

Planning for Now— and the Future

This book is about living well with HIV/AIDS by taking charge of day-to-day problems and challenges and coming up with ways to solve them. Whether your problem is getting used to a new medicine, starting an exercise routine, or dealing with the death of someone you love, the principles are the same. In this chapter we discuss some of the big questions people often have trouble thinking about. These questions tend to be about sensitive and sometimes unmentionable aspects of life: sex, grief, becoming dependent, money, and death. We touch on each of them here, and offer some suggestions that you may find useful.

The future can be frightening for people with HIV/AIDS. The most common way that people deal with their fear about the future is to not deal with it. People with illness often put off doing or thinking about the future, because they find it depressing or feel that there's nothing they can do to make any difference. Of course, if you think that nothing you do will make a difference, then you probably won't do anything, and your prediction will come true. Although there are many things to be concerned about—including loss of sex and intimacy, disability, loss of independence, money problems, and even death—there are also ways to approach these issues that will help you keep from feeling overwhelmed.

DOES MY ILLNESS MEAN AN END TO SEX AND INTIMACY?

Having HIV/AIDS should not redefine a person as an asexual being who's lost interest in sex. A person who has to face and adapt to changes caused by a chronic disease needs the love and comfort of close, intimate relationships perhaps more than ever. However, this aspect of life is often ignored, denied, or feared. For one thing, people with HIV/AIDS are rightly concerned about the risk that they will spread HIV to others. After all, even those who take potent "cocktail" HIV medications can still spread the disease. Learning to practice safer sex is necessary, but it's hard. Sometimes it seems easier just not to bother with sex. In Chapter 1, "Overview of HIV/AIDS Self-Management," we discuss practical advice about reducing risks during sexual activity. Sometimes HIV/AIDS itself can lead to lower hormone levels and decreased sex drive. Some people worry that the exertion of having sex will make them weaker. People with breathing problems worry that sex may be too strenuous and may bring on an attack of coughing and wheezing, or worse. Some people worry about starting new relationships, be they casual or more enduring. They struggle with whether to disclose their HIV status and wonder when is the right time to tell others.

One of the most subtle and devastating barriers to fulfilling sexuality is the damage that HIV/AIDS may cause to your self-image and self-esteem. You may believe you are physically unattractive as a result of your disease or medication side effects—for example, because of lipodystrophy, shortness of breath, weight loss, or a sense of not really being a whole, functioning being. This may cause you to avoid sexual situations, and to "try not to think about it."

Attitude and communication are the keys to resuming the sexual aspect of your relationships. You must believe that sex is a necessary and rewarding part of your life, and you must communicate this to your partner.

At present, there are few instructional materials on sexuality written specifically for people with physical disabilities. However, a number of very useful how-to guides are in bookstores, written for those wanting to enhance their sexual relationships. If you understand and appreciate your own needs and preferences and those of your partner, you can use creativity in adapting the activities described in these guides to your own relationship. It is important to avoid any assumption that there is only one "right way" to be sexually fulfilled.

Here are some ways to help you enhance sexual fulfillment:

- *Talk about your HIV status.* Your partner or potential partner needs to know. The sooner you talk about it, the sooner you can move on to healthy, enjoyable, safer sex practices.

- *Learn how to avoid spreading HIV when you have sex.* Your local HIV/AIDS service organization has programs to teach you how to have sex in ways that are as safe as possible for you and for others. Many have "Prevention for Positives" programs that are very helpful.

- *Try to establish a calm and relaxed atmosphere.* Stressful or highly emotional conversations tend to cause anxiety and are not conducive to satisfying sexual activity.

- *Find activities and positions that are safer, but also fun and comfortable for both of you.* Try to achieve open communication with your partner about what you like and want in the course of sexual activity.

- *Avoid sexual activity when you feel really tired.*

- *Avoid sexual activity right after a big meal.*

- *Avoid drinking alcohol before sex.*

- *If you have trouble with sexual performance, check with your doctor* to see if you are taking medication that may be the cause. Adjusting your dosage or switching to another medication may help.

- *Keep physically fit.* Being fit enhances sexual performance.

- *Get away* to enjoy a romantic weekend.

- *Consult a professional experienced in sexual counseling* if you are having chronic problems with arousal or a chronic loss of interest in sex. Short-term problems are often caused by depression.

GRIEVING: A NORMAL REACTION TO BAD NEWS

When we experience any kind of loss—small (such as losing a favorite possession) or large (such as losing a life partner or facing a disabling or terminal illness)—we go through an emotional process of grieving and coming to terms with the loss. A person with a chronic, disabling health problem experiences a variety of losses—loss of confidence, loss of self-esteem, loss of independence, loss of lifestyle, and—perhaps most painful of all—loss of positive self-image if the health problem has affected their physical appearance.

Elisabeth Kübler-Ross, who has written extensively about the grief process, describes its stages as follows:

- *Shock,* when we feel both mental and physical reactions to the initial recognition of the loss.

- *Denial,* when we tell ourselves, "No, it can't be true," and proceed to act for a time as though it were not true.

- *Anger,* when we ask, "Why me?" and search for someone or something to blame. ("If the doctor had diagnosed it earlier, I would've been cured," or "The job caused me too much stress.")

- *Bargaining,* when we say to ourselves, to someone else, or to God, "I'll never smoke again . . . ," or "I'll follow my treatment regimen absolutely to the letter . . . ," or "I'll go to church every Sunday . . . if only I can get over this."

- *Depression,* when real awareness sets in, we fully confront the truth about our situation, and experience deep feelings of sadness and hopelessness.

- *Acceptance,* when we eventually recognize that we must deal with what has happened, and make up our minds to do what we have to do.

We do not pass through these stages in linear, out-of-one and into-the-next fashion. We are more apt to have several, or even many, flip-flops back and forth between them. Don't be discouraged if you find yourself angry or depressed again, just when you thought you had reached acceptance. Many people get stuck at the anger and depression stages of the grief process. However, as we discussed in Chapter 10, "Using Your Mind to Manage Symptoms," there are several ways to move beyond these stages and toward acceptance.

WHAT IF I CAN'T TAKE CARE OF MYSELF ANYMORE?

Becoming helpless and dependent is the most basic fear among people who have potentially disabling health problems. This fear usually has physical as well as financial, social, and emotional components.

Physical Concerns of Day-to-Day Living

Nowadays people with HIV/AIDS are staying healthy, and living long, full lives by getting good health care and medications. This means that people with HIV are now living into old age and facing the same problems faced by everyone else who ages.

As your condition changes over time, you may need to consider changing your living situation. This change may involve hiring someone to help you in your home or moving to a living environment where help is provided. The decision about which alternative is best will be related to your needs and how they can best be met.

The first thing you will need to do is carefully *evaluate what you can do for yourself* and what activities of daily living will require some kind of help. These activities include the everyday things like getting out of bed, bathing, dressing, preparing and eating meals, cleaning house, shopping, and paying bills. Most people can do all of these—even though they may do them more slowly—with some modification or with some help from gadgets.

Some people, though, may eventually find that they are no longer able to do some of these activities without help from someone else. For example, you may still be able to fix meals, but your mobility may be impaired to the degree that grocery shopping is no longer possible. Or, if you have problems with fainting or sudden bouts of unconsciousness, you may need to have someone around at all times.

When you have analyzed your situation, make a list. In one column, list the activities you need help with; in another column, list ideas on what kind of help you might look for. For example:

WHEN YOU NEED HELP	
Need Help with	**What Kind of Help to Look for**
Can't go shopping	• Get friend to shop for me • Find volunteer shopping service • Shop on Internet or at store that delivers • Ask neighbor to shop for me when she does her own shopping • Get home-delivered meals
Can't be by myself	• Hire around-the-clock aide • Move in with relative or friend • Get "life-line" emergency response system • Move to board-and-care home • Move into shared-housing community or group home for people with HIV/AIDS

When you have listed your problems and their possible solutions, select the solution that seems the most workable, acceptable, and least expensive for your needs.

The selection should depend upon your finances, family and other resources you can call on, and how well the potential solutions will in fact solve your problem. Sometimes one solution will be the answer for several problems. For instance, if you can't shop and can't be alone, and chores are reaching the point of a foreseeable need for help, you may consider that an assisted-living environment or group home will solve all these problems, because it offers assistance with meals, regular housecleaning, and transportation for errands and medical appointments.

Even if you are not of "retirement" age, check policies; many facilities accept younger people. Most facilities for the retired take residents as young as 50, or younger if one member of a couple is the minimum age. If you are a young person, check with your local center for persons with disabilities or independent living center for direction to an out-of-home care facility that is appropriate for you.

Your appraisal of your situation and needs may well be aided by sitting down with a trusted friend or relative and discussing your abilities and limitations. Sometimes another person can spot things that we ourselves overlook, or would like to ignore.

Make changes in your life slowly and incrementally. You don't need to change your whole life around to solve one problem. Remember, too, that you can always change your mind, provided you don't "burn your bridges behind you." If you think that moving out of your own place to another living arrangement is the thing to do, don't give up your present home until you are settled into your new one and are sure you want to stay there. If you think you need help with some activities, hiring help at home is less drastic than moving out, and may suit your needs for quite a while. If you can't be alone and you live with a family member who is away during the day, attending programs at an adult or senior day care center may be enough to keep you safe and comfortable while your family is away. In fact, adult day care centers are ideal places to find new friends and activities geared to your abilities.

Several kinds of professionals can be of great help in giving you ideas about how to deal with your care needs:

- A *social worker* at your AIDS organization, center for persons with disabilities, or hospital social services department can be very helpful with decisions about financial and living arrangement problems, and with locating appropriate community resources. Some social workers are also trained in counseling persons with disabilities in emotional and relationship problems that may be associated with your health problem.

- A *licensed occupational therapist* can assess your daily living needs and suggest assistive devices or rearrangements in your environment to make life easier.

- An *attorney* should be on your "must see" list to help you set your financial affairs in order and preserve your assets, prepare a proper will, and perhaps execute a durable power of attorney for both health care and financial management. If finances are a concern, ask your local AIDS organization for the names of attorneys who offer free or reduced-cost services. Your local bar association or legal aid society can also refer you to attorneys who are competent in this area.

FINDING IN-HOME HELP

If you find that you cannot manage your daily activities alone, your first option is usually to hire someone to help. Most people just need a person called a *home aide*, or similar title. Home aides provide no medically related services that require licensing, but can help with bathing, dressing, meal preparation, and household chores.

You can find in-home help in a number of ways:

- *Home care agencies* are the easiest, but most expensive, way to find home care. You will usually find them listed under "home care" or "home nursing" in the telephone directory yellow pages. Such agencies are usually (but not always) private, for-profit businesses that supply caregiver staff to private individuals at home. The fees charged vary with the skill and license of the caregiver and will include amounts for Social Security, insurance, bonding, and profit for the agency. The fees are usually about double what you would expect to pay for someone you hire directly. If you can afford it, the advantage to hiring agency staff is that the agency assumes all payroll responsibilities, including Social Security and federal and state taxes; responsibility for the skill and integrity of the attendant; and immediate replacement of an ill or no-show attendant. The agency pays the staff directly. The client has no involvement with paying the attendant, but pays the agency.

- *Registered nurses* (RNs) hired through an agency are very expensive, but it is rare for home care for a chronically ill person to require a registered nurse. *Licensed vocational nurses* (LVNs) cost somewhat less, but are still expensive and are not usually needed unless nursing services are required (such as dressing changes, injections, ventilator management, etc.). *Certified nursing assistants* (CNAs) have some basic training in nursing, are much less expensive, and can provide satisfactory in-home care for any but the most critically ill person. Most agencies supply *home aides* as well as licensed staff. Unless you are bedridden or require some procedure that must be done by someone with a certain license, a home aide is probably the most appropriate for your needs.

- *Registries* supply prescreened lists from which you select the attendant or caregiver you wish to hire. You will be charged a placement fee, usually equal to one month's pay of the person hired. The agency will assume no liability for the skill or honesty of the people on its list, so you need to check references and interview carefully, just as you would someone who comes from any other source. This resource can be found in the yellow pages listed under "home nursing agencies," "home health services," or "registries." Some agencies provide both their own staff and registries of staff for you to select from.

- *Senior centers and centers serving persons with disabilities* may also provide links to home help. They often have listings of people who have called to say they are looking for home attendant work or who have posted a notice on the center's bulletin board. These job seekers are not screened, so you will need to interview them carefully and check their references before hiring.

- The *classified "employment wanted" section of your local newspaper* can be another good resource for experienced home care attendants. Because their patients usually progress to the need for more or sometimes less care than the attendant was hired to provide, these aides' jobs are by nature temporary, and they are often looking for a new placement. You can find a competent helper through the newspaper, but the advice to interview carefully is valid here, too.

- *Word of mouth* is probably your best source of help. Talk to someone who has employed a helper, or who knows of an aide who has worked for an acquaintance. Putting the word out through your family and social network may result in a jewel.

- *Home sharing* may be a solution if you have space and can offer lodging to someone in exchange for help. This arrangement works best if you need help mainly with household and garden chores. However, you may find a helper willing to provide personal care such as help with dressing, bathing, and meal preparation. Some communities have agencies or government bureaus that help home sharers and home sharees locate each other.

FINDING OUT-OF-HOME CARE

If getting the care you need just isn't possible in your own home, it may be time to think about moving someplace where you can be safe and comfortable. Here are some of the options to look into.

Residential Care Homes

Residential care homes, or *board-and-care homes,* are licensed by state or county social services agencies. They provide nonmedical care and supervision for persons who cannot live alone. These homes fall into two categories: large and small. The small ones have about six "residents," who live in a family-like setting in a neighborhood residence. The large ones have more residents, sometimes hundreds, who live in a boarding house or hotel-like setting. They take meals in a central dining room and have individual or shared rooms, with activities taking place in large common rooms.

In either type of facility, the services to the residents are the same—all meals, assistance with bathing and dressing as needed, laundry, housekeeping, transportation to medical appointments, supervision, and assistance with taking medications. Larger facilities usually have professional activities directors. Residents of the larger facilities usually need to be more independent, since there is generally not as much personal attention as in the smaller homes.

These homes are licensed in most states for residents who are either "elderly" (over 62) or "adult" (under 62). The adult category is further divided into facilities for residents with mental illness, residents with mental retardation, and residents with physical disabilities.

It is important when considering a residential care home to evaluate the nature of the persons already living there to make sure you will fit in. For example, some of these facilities may cater to individuals who are mentally confused. If you are mentally clear, you would not find much companionship there. If everyone is hard of hearing, you might find conversation tiring.

Although all homes are required by law to provide wholesome meals, you should make sure the cuisine is to your liking and meets your dietary needs. If you need a vegetarian or diabetic diet, for instance, be sure the operator is willing to prepare your special meals.

Monthly fees for residential care homes vary, depending on whether they are spartan or luxurious. The monthly cost of the most spartan facilities is about the same as the monthly SSI (Supplemental Security Income) benefit. They accept SSI beneficiaries and bill the government directly. The more luxurious the home with respect to furnishings, neighborhood, services, and so on, the greater the cost. Even the nicest of these will probably cost less than full-time, twenty-four-hour, seven-day in-home care.

Skilled Nursing Facilities

Sometimes called *nursing homes* or *convalescent hospitals, skilled nursing facilities* provide the most comprehensive care for severely ill or disabled people. If you have PCP or toxoplasmosis, you may need to be transferred from an acute hospital to a skilled nursing facility for a period of rehabilitation before going home.

No care situation seems to inspire more fear than the prospect of going to a nursing home. "Horror stories" in the news media help to foster the anxiety about what awful fate will befall anyone who has the misfortune to have to go to one. However, public scrutiny is valuable in helping to ensure that standards of care and humane and competent treatment are provided. It must be remembered that nursing homes serve a critical need. When you really need a nursing home, there is usually no other care situation that will meet your need.

Skilled nursing facilities provide medically related care for people who are no longer able to be in a nonmedical care situation. For example, you may need intravenous or injected medications that must be administered or monitored by professional nursing staff. Or you may be very physically limited and need help getting in and out of bed, eating, bathing, or dealing with bladder or bowel control. Skilled nursing facilities can also manage care of feeding tubes, respirators, and other high-tech care equipment. If you are only partially or temporarily disabled, you may need a skilled nursing facility for physical, occupational, or speech therapy; wound care; or other therapies.

Not all nursing homes provide all types of care. Some specialize in rehabilitation and therapies, and some specialize in long-term custodial care. Some provide high-tech nursing services; others do not.

In selecting a nursing home, you should seek the help of the *hospital discharge planner* or *social worker,* or a similar professional from a home care agency or center for persons with disabilities. There are organizations that monitor local nursing homes. Each nursing home is required by law to post in a prominent place the name and phone number of the "ombudsman," the person assigned by the state licensing agency to assist patients and their families with problems in relation to their nursing home care. The agencies that can help you with this are listed in the yellow pages under "social service organizations."

Hospice

Although it isn't for everyone, hospice care is an important option that everyone should at least know about. Hospice philosophy is based on the belief that death is part of life and is something we will all experience. Therefore, hospice care concentrates on relieving pain and supporting emotional and spiritual needs. Hospice care doesn't emphasize prolonging life as long as is medically possible. Instead, the individual is given an environment to reflect on life and develop a sense of peace. The hope is that with good hospice care, a person can meet the end more peacefully than might otherwise be possible.

Many communities have excellent hospice facilities where people with serious illnesses can live and be cared for during the final stage of life. Hospice care can often be provided in your own home, too. The best way to find out about hospice care is through your local AIDS service organization or through your medical care site.

WILL I HAVE ENOUGH MONEY
TO PAY FOR MY CARE?

Next to the basic fear of physical dependency, the greatest fear of most people with serious illness is not having enough money to pay for their needs. Being sick often requires expensive care and treatment. If you are too ill or disabled to work, the loss of income and health insurance coverage may present an overwhelming financial burden. You can, however, avoid some of the risks by planning ahead and knowing your resources. There are a number of government benefit programs you should know about.

- *Social Security.* If you are too sick to work—either permanently or for some extended period—you may be entitled to draw Social Security on the basis of your disability. People with symptomatic HIV infection may be able to qualify for disability by showing that they have had one or more illnesses—such as *Pneumocystis* pneumonia (PCP), toxoplasmosis, or another AIDS-related condition. People who haven't had one of these illnesses may have to obtain other documentation to qualify. If you qualify and have dependent children, they also would receive Social Security benefits. If you have been disabled for a specified period (as of this writing, two years), you may be entitled to Medicare coverage for your medical treatment needs.

- *Medicaid* and *SSI (Supplemental Security Income).* If you have only minimal savings and little or no income, the federal Medicaid program can pay for medical treatment and long-term skilled or custodial care. The eligibility rules on assets and income differ from state to state. If you have savings of less than the U.S. median of one month's wages, and income at or slightly above the official federal "poverty line" (which changes from year to year), you should consult your local social services department to see whether you are entitled to benefits. If Social Security benefits are unavailable or insufficient, the Supplemental Security Income (SSI) program is available to those who meet the same eligibility criteria as for Medicaid.

If you have some savings, you will have to pay for your care until you have "spent down" to meet the asset limitation criteria for Medicaid and

SSI. If you have income above a certain level, you will be responsible for what is termed a "co-payment," or "share-of-cost," which you must pay before Medicaid will begin to supplement.

The social work department in the hospital where you have been treated can advise you about your own situation and eligibility for these programs. Your local agency serving persons with disabilities also usually has benefits counselors and advisors who can refer you to programs and resources for which you may be eligible. Local AIDS and community service organizations often have benefits counselors who are knowledgeable about the ins and outs of health care insurance.

Be warned: Although the government can provide a helpful (and in cases, lifesaving) safety net, dealing with government agencies is difficult. Be patient, don't be surprised if you run into problems, and even if you are turned down, keep at it.

I NEED HELP, BUT I DON'T WANT HELP—NOW WHAT?

We all emerge from childhood reaching for and cherishing every possible form of independence—the driver's license, the first job, the first checking account, the first time we go out and don't have to tell anyone where we're going or when we'll be back, and so on. In these and many other ways, we demonstrate to ourselves and to others that we are in charge of our lives and able to take care of ourselves without any help from parents.

If a time comes when we must face the realization that we need help—that we can no longer manage completely on our own—it may seem like we are making a return to childhood, having to let someone else be in charge of our lives. This dependency can be very painful and embarrassing. Some people in this situation become depressed and can no longer find any joy in life. Others fight off the recognition of their need for help, possibly placing themselves in danger and making life difficult and frustrating for those who would like to be helpful. Some people give up completely and expect others to take total responsibility for their lives, demanding attention and services from their partners, friends, and family. If you are having one or more of these reactions, you can help yourself feel better and develop a more positive response.

The message in the "Serenity Prayer"—". . . *grant me the serenity to accept the things I cannot change; the courage to change the things I can; and the wisdom to know the difference*"—is fundamental to staying in charge of your life. You must be able to correctly evaluate your situation. You must identify those activities that require the help of someone else (going shopping or cleaning house, for instance) and those activities you can still do on your own (getting dressed, paying bills, writing letters). This means making decisions, and as long as you keep the decision-making prerogative, you are in charge. It is important to make a decision and take action while you are still able to, before circumstances intervene and the decision gets made for you. This means being realistic and honest with yourself.

There are several approaches you can take to get help and still stay in charge of your life:

- *Talk with a sympathetic listener,* either a professional counselor or a sensible, close friend or family member. An objective listener often helps by pointing out alternatives and options that you may have overlooked or were not aware of. Such a person can provide information or another point of view or interpretation of a situation that you would not have come upon yourself. This is part of the self-management process. Be very careful, however, in evaluating advice from someone who has something to sell you. There are many people whose solution to your problem just happens to be whatever it is they are selling—health or burial insurance policies, special furniture, "sunshine cruises," special magazines, or health foods with curative properties.

- *Be as open and reasonable as you can be* when talking with family members or friends who offer to be helpful. At the same time, try to make them understand that you will reserve for yourself the right to decide how much and what kind of help you will accept. They will probably be more cooperative and understanding if you say, "Yes, I do need some help with . . . , but I still want to do . . . myself."

- *Insist on being consulted.* Lay the ground rules with your helpers early on. Ask to be presented with choices, so that you can decide what is best for you, as you see it. If you try to objectively weigh the suggestions made to you and don't dismiss every option out of hand, people will consider you able to make reasonable decisions and will continue to provide you the opportunity to do so.

- *Be appreciative.* Recognize the goodwill and efforts of those who want to help. Even though you may be embarrassed, you will maintain your dignity by accepting with grace the help that is offered, if you need it. If you are truly convinced that you are being offered help you don't need, you can decline it with tact and appreciation. For example, say, "I appreciate your offer to have Thanksgiving dinner at your house, but I'd like to continue having it here. I could really use some help, though—maybe with the cleanup after dinner."

- *Consult a professional counselor* if you are consistently unable to come to terms with your increasing need to depend on others for help in managing your living situation. This should be someone who has experience with the emotional and social issues of people with disabling health problems. Your local agency for providing services to persons with disabilities should be able to refer you to the right kind of counselor. The local or national organization dedicated to serving people with HIV/AIDS can also refer you to support groups and classes to help you in dealing with your condition. You should be able to locate the agency you need through the telephone book yellow pages under the listing, "social service organizations."

We need to be sure that we do reach out to family and friends and ask for the help we need when we recognize that we can't go on alone. It sometimes happens that, expecting rejection, people fail to ask for help. Some people try to hide their need in fear that their need will cause loved ones to withdraw. Families often complain, "If we'd only known . . ." when they learn that a loved one had needs for help that went unmet.

If you really cannot turn to close family or friends because they are unable or unwilling to become involved in your care, there are agencies dedicated to providing for such situations. Through your local social service department's adult protective services program or family services association, you should be able to locate a case manager who will be able to organize the resources in your community to provide the help you need. The social services department in your local hospital can also put you in touch with the right agency.

I'M AFRAID OF DEATH

Fear of death is something most of us begin to experience only when something happens to bring us face-to-face with the possibility of our own death. Losing someone close, surviving an accident that could have been fatal, or learning about a health condition that may shorten our life usually causes us to consider the inevitability of our own passing. Many people, even then, try to avoid facing the future because they are afraid to think about it.

If you are ready to think about your own future—about the imminent or distant prospect that your life will most certainly end—then the ideas that follow will be useful to you. If you are not ready to think about it just yet, put this section aside and come back to it later.

Getting Your House in Order

The most useful way to come to terms with your eventual death is to take positive steps to prepare for it. This means "getting your house in order" by attending to all the small and large details that are necessary. If you continue to avoid dealing with these details, you will create problems for yourself and for those who will become involved with your situation in a significant way. There are several components to getting your house in order:

- *Decide and convey to others your wishes about how and where you want to be during your last days and hours.* Do you want to be in a hospital or at home? When do you want life-prolonging procedures stopped? At what point do you want to let nature take its course when it is determined that death is inevitable? Who should be with you—only the few who are nearest and dearest, or all the people you care about and want to see one last time? See Chapter 15, "Making Your Wishes Known," for more information about communicating this information to family, friends, and caregivers.

- *Make a will.* Even if your estate is a small one, you may have definite preferences about who should have what. If you have a large estate, the tax implications of a proper will may be very significant.

- *Make arrangements—or at least plans—for your funeral.* Your grieving family will be relieved not to have to decide what you would want and how much to spend. There are prepaid "future need" funeral plans available, and you can purchase burial space of the type you prefer.

- *Prepare an advance directive* (see Chapter 15) and a durable power of attorney that will let someone manage your financial affairs. You should discuss your health care wishes with your personal physician, even if he or she doesn't seem to be very interested. (Your physician may also have trouble facing the prospect of losing you.) Be sure to include some kind of document or notation in your medical records that indicates your wishes in case you can't communicate them when the time comes.

- *Be sure that the persons who you want to handle things after your death are aware of all that they need to know*—your wishes, your plans and arrangements, and the location of necessary documents. You will need to talk to them, or at least prepare a detailed letter of instruction and give it to someone who can be counted on to deliver it to the proper person when necessary. You may not want your spouse or partner to have to take on such things as funeral responsibilities, but he or she may be the best person to keep your letter of instruction and know when to give it to your designated agent. You can purchase at any well-stocked stationery store a preorganized kit in which to place a copy of your will and durable power of attorney, other important papers, and information about your financial and personal affairs. This kit also contains forms to fill out about bank and charge accounts, insurance policies, the location of important documents, your safe-deposit box and where the key is kept, and so on. This is a handy, concise way of getting together everything that anyone may need to know about.

- *"Finish business" with the world around you.* Mend your relationships. Pay your debts, both financial and personal. Say what needs to be said to those who need to hear it. Do what needs to be done. Forgive yourself. Forgive others.

- *Share your feelings about your death.* Most family and close friends are reluctant to initiate such a conversation but appreciate it if you bring it up. You may find that there is much to say to and hear from your loved ones. If you find that they are unwilling to listen to you talk about your death, find someone who will be comfortable and empathic in listening to you. Your partner, family, and friends may be able to listen to you later on. Remember, those who love you will also go through the stages of grieving when they have to think about the prospect of losing you.

DYING

A large component in the fear of death is fear of the unknown. "What will it be like?" "Will it be painful?" "What will happen to me after I die?"

Most people who die of a disease are ready to die when the time comes. Painkillers and the disease process itself weaken the body and mind, and the awareness of self diminishes without the realization that this is happening. Most people just "slip away," with the transition between the state of living and that of no longer living barely identifiable. Reports from people who have been "brought back to life" after being in a state of "clinical death" indicate that they experienced a sense of peacefulness and clarity and were not frightened.

However, a dying person may sometimes feel very lonely and abandoned. Regrettably, many people cannot deal with their own emotions when they are around a person they know to be dying and so deliberately avoid that person's company, or they may engage in superficial chitchat, broken by awkward silences. This is often puzzling and hurtful to the dying person, who needs companionship and solace.

You can help by telling your partner, family, and friends what you want and need from them—attention, entertainment, comfort, practical help, and so on. Again, when people have something positive to do, they are better able to cope with their emotions. If you can engage your loved ones in specific activities, they can feel needed and can relate to you around the activity. This will give you something to talk about, occupy time, or at least provide a definition of the situation for them and for you.

Again, if you choose to die at home, a hospice can be very helpful. Hospice organizations provide both physical and emotional care for people who are dying, and for their families.

SUGGESTED READING

Callanan, Maggie, and Kelley, Patricia. *Final Gifts: Understanding the Special Awareness, Needs, and Communications of the Dying*. New York: Bantam Books, 1997.

Copeland, Mary Ellen, and McKay, Matthew. *The Depression Workbook: A Guide for Living with Depression and Manic Depression*. 2nd ed. Oakland, Calif.: New Harbinger Publications, 2002.

Kübler-Ross, Elisabeth. *Living with Death and Dying*. Indianapolis, Ind.: Macmillan, 1997.

Leslie, Mark. *Dying with AIDS: Living with AIDS*. Winnipeg, Canada. The Muses' Company, 1993.

Lewinsohn, Peter. *Control Your Depression*. Revised ed. New York: Simon & Schuster, 1992.

Longaker, Christine. *Facing Death and Finding Hope: A Guide to the Emotional and Spiritual Care of the Dying*. New York: Doubleday, 1998.

New York State Department of Health. *There's Something I Need to Tell You: A Step-by-Step Guide to Telling Your Partner that They May Have HIV* at http://www.aids-ed.org/pdf/p02-et/et-05-00/tellyou.pdf. Accessed August 31, 2005. (Spanish language version available at http://www.aids-ed.org/pdf/p02-et/et-05-00/tellyou_spanish.pdf)

Project Inform. *Sex and Prevention Concerns for Positive People* at http://www.projectinform.org/pdf/sex.pdf. Accessed August 31, 2005.

CHAPTER SEVENTEEN

Finding Resources

A major part of becoming a self-manager of your HIV/AIDS is knowing when you need help and how to find help. Seeking help to perform daily tasks and chores or to assist with other aspects of your life does *not* mean that you have fallen victim to your illness. Rather, knowing where to go for help with specific aspects of your life takes initiative—evaluation of your condition and your own capabilities. By becoming more aware of the symptoms you experience throughout the day, you can better predict the amount of energy and patience you will have to accomplish tasks. If you find that you come up short on energy, time, patience, or capability for some tasks, you can evaluate where help from other resources will preserve your own resources for those things most important to you.

The first resource you will probably turn to for help is *family* or *close friends*. Some find it difficult, however, to ask for help from people they know. Finding the right words to ask for help is discussed in Chapter 14, "Communicating." Unfortunately, some people either do not have family or close friends to call on or cannot bring themselves to ask. If this is the case, you must look for other resources in your community. This chapter shows you how to search for resources, and lists some of the most useful sources for the kind of help and information commonly needed by people with HIV/AIDS.

GETTING STARTED: FINDING CLUES AND NETWORKING

Finding resources in your community is a little like a treasure hunt: Creative thinking will help you win the game. Finding what you need may be as simple as looking in the telephone book and making a couple of phone calls. Other times, you will need to follow clues, and possibly start all over again when the clue leads to a dead end.

Where do you start? Suppose you find it difficult to prepare meals because prolonged standing is too tiring or painful. After some thought, you decide that you want to continue cooking for yourself rather than have someone else cook your meals. The next step, then, is to explore the prospect of having your kitchen altered so you can prepare meals from a seated position. Where can you find an architect or contractor who has knowledge of and experience in kitchen alterations for people with physical limitations? Looking at the yellow pages and the classified section of the newspaper reveals pages of ads and listings for architects and contractors; some say they specialize in kitchens, while others don't mention any specialty. None mentions anything about designing for physical limitations. A couple of phone calls to contractors listing kitchens as a specialty are unsuccessful in finding anyone experienced in kitchens for persons with physical limitations.

Now what? You could call every business listed until you find what you need. Not only would this be time-consuming, but you may not feel comfortable hiring a given contractor until you talk to someone who personally knows this person's work. Here is where creative thought and networking enter the picture. Who else do you know who may have information of this kind? Maybe someone who works with people with disabilities would have ideas—an occupational or physical therapist, your local AIDS service organization, your city or county's human services department or commission, the nearest independent living center for persons with disabilities, the community college disabilities services office, or an orthopedic supply store. You may talk to someone who doesn't have the answer but says, "Gosh, Jack So-and-So just had his kitchen remodeled to accommodate his wheelchair.

Maybe he can help you find someone." Jack is probably a great lead to follow. He may be able to give you not only the name of a contractor who can do the work, but also some ideas about cost and other concerns before you go any further in the process. Jack has probably done much of the groundwork already and can save you time and trouble.

Suppose your search still isn't successful. Every community has people who are natural resources. These "naturals" seem to know everyone and know where everything is. They tend to be folks who have lived in the community a long time and have been involved in it. They are natural problem solvers—the community members people always seek out for advice. If you were to call such a person, he or she would probably know the answer or could set you on the right path to get the answer. This "natural" could be a friend, a business associate, the mail carrier, your physician, your pet's veterinarian, the checker at the corner grocery, the pharmacist, the bus or taxi driver, a real estate agent, the chamber of commerce receptionist, or the librarian. All you need to do is think of this person as an information resource.

RESOURCES FOR RESOURCES

Most searches for information begin with a single step and expand into a web of networking that will bring you into contact with unexpected resources. The following list will give you many starting points for finding the resources you need:

- *The telephone book* is where most people start to look for community resources. Particularly if you need to hire someone to do something for you, you should check the telephone book for extensive listings of people and organizations ready to help you.

- *Local HIV/AIDS information and referral services* are listed in your telephone book. Look under "AIDS information and referral" (or "HIV information and referral"), "United Way information and referral," or simply "information and referral" in your county or city government listings. Once you have an information and referral telephone number, your searches become much easier. These services maintain a huge file of referral addresses and telephone numbers for just about any kind of help you may need. Even if they don't have the answer to your immediate need, they will almost always be able to refer you to another agency that can speed along your search.

- *Voluntary agencies dedicated to your disease* are one of the most important resources for either information or help. For people with HIV/AIDS, this means your local AIDS foundation. Agencies of this type are funded by contributions from individuals and corporate sponsors and provide up-to-date information about your disease as well as support and direct services to people with AIDS. You can become a member of these organizations, which entitles you to receive regular bulletins by mail. You do not, however, have to be a member to qualify for their services. They are here to serve you.

- *National HIV/AIDS organizations* maintain telephone hotlines to offer information about all kinds of resources, many of which may be available in your community.

- *HIV/AIDS resource guides* are often published by local HIV/AIDS organizations and provide information about services and resources available to people with HIV/AIDS. The listings are categorized by type—financial, medical, social, and mental health and support—and are updated regularly.

- *Other community organizations, such as community centers and religious social service agencies,* also offer information and referral services as well as direct services. The latter may include classes, recreational opportunities, nutrition programs, legal and tax help, and social programs. There is probably a community center close to you. An employee in your city government or local librarian will know where they are, and the calendar section of your newspaper usually has information about programs these organizations offer.

- *Religious groups* usually offer information and social services to those in need, either directly through the local church, synagogue, or mosque, or through the Council of Churches, Catholic Charities, Islamic center, or Jewish social service groups. To get help from religious organizations, start with your local church, synagogue, or mosque; they will help you or refer you to someone who can help. You need not be a member of the religion or of its local organization to receive help.

- *Hospital and health care organizations* may also offer services. Many clinics caring for people with HIV/AIDS have access to excellent social workers and case managers who can give you much help. Call your local hospital, clinic, or health insurance plan and ask for their social service department. *Your doctor* will also be aware of the services available in the health care organizations he or she is affiliated with.

- *Public libraries* are invaluable resources, particularly when you are looking for information about your disease. The library, and the *reference librarian* in particular, can serve as an information and referral service as well. Often the reference section of the library has a gem of a book or pamphlet that lists the resources you are looking for. The reference librarian can probably take you right to it—and perhaps show you others as well. Even if you think you are good at library research, it's a good idea to ask the reference librarian if you may have overlooked something. Reference librarians see volumes of material cross their desks and are knowledgeable about community resources.

  Libraries are often equipped with public computer terminals, so even if you don't own your own computer, you can still probably access the Internet at the library.

- *University and college libraries* are also open to the general public. In fact, the regional *government documents* sections of these libraries are required by law to be open to the public at no charge. Government publications have been written about just about any subject, and the health-related publications are particularly extensive. You can find information on everything from organic gardening to detailed nutritional recipes. The librarians are usually very helpful, and these publications are "your tax dollars at work."

- *Medical school libraries*—if you are fortunate enough to have one in your community—are another resource for information (although they are not a place to look for help with tasks). As you would expect, a great deal of information about disease and treatment is found at a medical library, but unless you have some special knowledge about medicine, the information you find there can be intimidating and confusing. Use medical libraries with care.

- The *"back matter" in books* can be another great resource. Look for the reading list (sometimes titled "Bibliography") and other resource lists at the back of a book related to your disease. This information may be easy to miss because it is found just before or after the index. The content in the back of a book is helpful for finding information as well as names and addresses of agencies and other organizations.

- *Local newspapers* are an excellent source of information. The health or science editor and the calendar-of-events editor can be very knowledge-able about community resources. Gay community newspapers in partic-ular contain a great deal of information. Two newspaper sections that can be most helpful in your search for resources are the *calendar-of-events section* and the *classified section*. Organizations advertise classes, lectures, and other events in both of these sections. In the classifieds, look under "Announcements," "Health," or any other heading that looks promis-ing (you'll find an index of the headings used by your newspaper print-ed at the front of the classified section). Even if you are not interested in the particular events advertised, the contact telephone numbers may be good leads in your search for something else. Look in other logical places for news stories that may be of interest, such as the pages around the cal-endar section or the health-and-fitness section (you might find an exer-cise program for people with your health problem there, for example).

- *The Internet* is an almost endless source of information about HIV/ AIDS. Of course, you must have access to a computer at home, work, or the library that is connected to the Internet (either by modem or directly linked), and you have to be comfortable using the computer. But if you can access it, the Internet can be a way to research treatment options, ask questions, learn about studies—all kinds of information. The great thing about the Internet is that literally everything is there. The not-so-great thing about the Internet is that . . . literally everything is there. Anyone can put anything on the Internet. No one edits the material, so the quality varies drastically.

So how does one separate what's valid from what's not (or from what's even crazy)? It can be hard to tell. Web sites created by official organizations such as the U.S. Centers For Disease Control (CDC), National Institutes of Health (NIH), universities, or the major AIDS organizations (such as Project Inform, Gay Men's Health Crisis, or thebody.com) are reliable, and they generally have material that's in the mainstream of thought about AIDS. Information from newsgroups or "personal" Web sites is often more interesting but you may need to treat much of it skeptically. People may try to sell you things—look out for extravagant claims about new "cures." Discuss things you've heard about on the Internet with others. If something sounds too good to be true, it probably is.

All of these resources are just first steps. Once you've started down any path, you'll find that with persistence and creativity, your information and support network will grow to give you many choices. You are not alone.

A REFERENCE GUIDE TO KEY HIV/AIDS RESOURCES

National Hotlines
National AIDS Hotline
(800) 342-2437
TTY (800) 243-7889

Operated by the Centers for Disease Control (CDC). Open 24 hours a day. Offers information, referrals to agencies, and trained counselors.

National Prevention Information Network (NPIN)
(800) 458-5231
TTY (800) 243-7012
e-mail: info@cdcnpin.org
Internet: www.cdcnpin.org

Provides access to all of the CDC's published information between 9 A.M. and 8 P.M. Eastern time, Monday through Friday. You can get referrals to AIDS organizations and services, order publications, get information about AIDS in the workplace, learn about the latest clinical trials, or use an automated service to get information via fax or e-mail. You can also order a free catalogue of HIV/AIDS education and prevention materials.

Internet Links

Things change quickly in the fields serving the HIV/AIDS community. The most up-to-date information resources for people with HIV/AIDS are probably on the Internet. Here are four Web sites that are excellent gateways to HIV/AIDS resources. Each has extensive links to more specific organizations and other resources.

HIVInSite (University of California, San Francisco)
http://hivinsite.ucsf.edu

The Body
www.thebody.com

Gay Men's Health Crisis
www.gmhc.org

Johns Hopkins AIDS Service
www.hopkins-aids.edu

Project Inform
www.projectinform.org

AEGIS (Sisters of St. Elizabeth of Hungary—updated hourly)
www.aegis.com

For information on pharmaceutical patient-assistance programs, with a search engine to find specific drugs, contact:

Association for Clinicians for the Underserved
www.clinicians.org
National Office
501 Darby Creek Road, Suite 20
Lexington, KY 40509-1606
Tel: (606) 263-0046
Fax: (606) 263-7580
e-mail: acu@clinicians.org

INDEX